Dysphagia
Cookbook

Nourishing Soft-Food Recipes for People With Difficulty Chewing and Swallowing | 28-Day Meal Plan Included

Audrey Robinson

Table of Contents

Introduction

Dysphagia is defined as a disorder of the swallow mechanism marked by difficulties in transferring liquids, solids, or both from the mouth to the stomach. When a person has dysphagia, they may experience pain when swallowing or have the sensation of food sticking in their throat. Dysphagia can make it difficult to eat or drink and can lead to weight loss or dehydration if left untreated. There are four levels of dysphagia diet, each of which has different restrictions on what types of food and liquids a person can consume.

A person with dysphagia may need to follow a diet that includes only soft foods or liquids, or they may need to avoid certain foods or liquids altogether. Each level of dysphagia has its own restrictions, so a person with dysphagia must consult with their doctor to determine the best diet for them.

In this cookbook, you'll find everything you need to know about this difficult swallowing disorder and how to follow a diet that is tailored to your level of dysphagia. It also includes 100 delicious and nourishing soft-food recipes and a 28-day meal plan, so a person with dysphagia can easily follow the recipes and avoid food allergies or intolerance problems.

If you or a loved one struggles with dysphagia, this book is a valuable resource for finding delicious and nutritious soft-food recipes. There's something for everyone in this cookbook so that you can enjoy delicious and nutritious food no matter your dietary restrictions.

Chapter 1

Understanding Dysphagia & The Diet You Should Follow

Dysphagia is a medical term that refers to difficulty swallowing. It is not a disease but a symptom of an underlying problem. The underlying problem could be a physical obstruction, such as a tumor, or a neurological condition, such as Parkinson's disease. Dysphagia can also be caused by psychological factors, such as anxiety or depression.

There are three types of dysphagia: oropharyngeal, esophageal, and mixed. People with oropharyngeal dysphagia have trouble getting food or liquid to go down the right way. Esophageal dysphagia happens when the muscles in the esophagus don't work right. Mixed dysphagia is a combination of the two. People with this type of dysphagia can't swallow either food or liquids properly.

The treatment varies depending on the cause of the dysphagia. If the cause is physical, such as a tumor, treatment may involve surgery to remove the obstruction. If the cause is neurological, such as Parkinson's disease, treatment may involve medications to improve muscle function. If the cause is psychological, such as anxiety or depression, treatment may involve therapy to address the underlying issue.

What Is A Dysphagia Diet

People with dysphagia may need to follow a special diet. The diet is designed to make swallowing easier. A dysphagia diet is needed because the muscles in the throat and mouth don't work the way they're supposed to. If you don't eat the right foods, your dysphagia will get worse. to follow because swallowing is difficult for people with the condition. The diet is broken down into four levels, and each level is designed to help a particular type of dysphagia. Each level is a little bit different, so you will need to talk to your doctor to find out which level you need to be on.

The Levels of Dysphagia Diet

A dysphagia diet is used to make eating and drinking easier for people who have trouble swallowing. It is a set of guidelines that help make sure you're getting the right nutrition while still being able to eat and drink safely. There are four levels of dysphagia diet, and each level has different restrictions.

Level 1 (Pureed): This is the most restrictive level of diet. All food should be pureed to avoid any risk of choking. All liquids should be thickened to avoid aspiration. This level is often used for people who have moderate to severe dysphagia with poor oral function and are not able to eat or drink.

Level 2 (Mechanical Altered): Foods and liquids must be mechanically altered, which means they must be cut, mixed, or stirred in a way that doesn't increase the risk of choking. There is more leeway at this level. Not all foods are pureed, but they must be soft-textured, well-cooked, minced, or mashed. This level is appropriate for patients with mild to moderate dysphagia and who can tolerate some textures.

Level 3 (Chopped and Moistened): Foods can be any texture, but they must be cut into small pieces and moistened to make them easier to swallow. Liquids can be any consistency, but they should be thickened if needed. This level is appropriate for patients with mild dysphagia who can tolerate all textures.

Level 4 (Normal/Regular): Foods and liquids can be in any form. However, they must be in normal or regular size and shape. This level is for patients who can swallow most foods and liquids without difficulty.

Chapter 2

Recommended Foods & Prohibited Foods As Per Patient Type

Dysphagia manifests itself in 4 levels of severity, classified according to the type of disorder and the stage of swallowing at which it occurs. For each, a specific diet is indicated, consisting of foods and beverages with characteristics appropriate to the patient's chewing and swallowing problems.

Patient type GRADE 1: Patients who are unable to chew and swallow

- Foods allowed: Homogeneous semi-liquid foods
- Liquids: Only if thickened
- To be avoided: Foods that shatter or crumble; Sticky foods.

Patient type GRADE 2: Patients with impaired chewing ability and severely impaired swallowing

- Foods allowed: Pureed foods (creamy or pureed consistency)
- Liquids: Preferably thickened
- To be avoided: Whole or chopped foods

Patient type GRADE 3: Patients with limited chewing and acceptable swallowing

- Foods allowed: Soft foods cooked, chopped or reduced to small pieces; no need for blending; remove tough or stringy parts; sauces or creams may be used to change texture.
- Liquids: Evaluate if tolerated.
- To be avoided: Raw foods, dry or crunchy foods, foods that melt in the mouth.

Patient type GRADE 4: Patients able to take foods that are easily chewed and swallowed

- Foods allowed: Soft, nonshake foods
  - remove the harder, fibrous or stringy parts
  - sauces or creams can be used to change the texture.
- Liquids: No a priori contraindications, but evaluate if tolerated.
- To be avoided: Raw foods; dry or crunchy foods; foods that melt in the mouth.

Chapter 3

General Foods To Eat & Foods To Avoid

Foods To Eat

SEMI-LIQUID FOODS:
- Ice creams (left to melt/soften at room temperature)
- Liquid creams
- Vegetable purees
- Smoothies, milkshakes and homogenized fruit, yogurt
- Tomato sauce

SEMI-SOLID FOODS:
- Thick purées and smoothies, creams
- Homogenized meat and fish
- Purees
- Soft-boiled eggs
- Puddings, panna cotta, creams, mousses
- Polenta
- Soft and creamy cheeses (cottage cheese, spreadable cheese, robiola...)

SOFT-SOLID FOODS:
- Well-cooked and well-seasoned pasta, stuffed pasta
- Meatballs, meatloaf
- Hard-boiled eggs
- Barbed fish
- Cooked non-starchy vegetables
- Banana and ripe fruit or cooked fruit
- Soufflé

Foods To Avoid

NO to foods with double consistency, this means solid and liquid consistency put together, because they have different chewing and/or sliding times in the palate and can cause swallowing problems for the person with dysphagia. Foods of this type are: *Minestrone with noodles, rice in broth, minestrone in pieces, fruit salad, juices or yogurt with pieces of fruit or cereal inside, milk with crumbled toast inside, chocolate with nuts...*

NO also to:
*   dried fruits
*   crunchy foods such as: Fried foods, potato chips, pretzels, toast, breadsticks
*   foods that crumble easily, whose crumbs can lead to choking: Puff pastry, bread crusts, pie crusts, cookies
*   candies, confections, nuts, peanuts, chewing gum, toffee
*   legumes and vegetable peels
*   fresh fruits with seeds: Currants, grapes, pomegranate, etc.
*   small-format pasta, rice, barley, wheat, cous-cous
*   acidic foods (citrus fruits)
*   stringy and stringy foods: Vegetables such as artichoke, fennel, green beans, the hard part of asparagus; fruits such as pineapple; stringy and stodgy meat;
*   stringy cheeses that can form a "Pudding" That is difficult to swallow (e.g., cooked mozzarella, tosella)
*   dumplings and sticky foods such as sandwich bread that may stick to the palate and not slide well
*   spicy foods
*   spirits

Breakfast

Lemony Grape Juice

 Prep Time: 10 minutes   Cooking Time: 0 minutes   Servings: 3

INGREDIENTS

4 cups seedless white grapes
2 tbsp fresh lemon juice

DIRECTIONS

1. Put all the fixings into your blender and pulse well. Strain the juice in a fine-mesh strainer in a bowl.
2. Gently press the pulp to extract all possible liquid, then discard it. Serve!

Nutrition: Calories: 141; Fat: 0.35g; Carbs: 37g; Protein: 1.49g

---

Cantaloupe-Mix Smoothie

 Prep Time: 5 minutes   Cooking Time: 0 minutes   Servings: 2

INGREDIENTS

1 cup cantaloupe, diced
½ cup mango, diced
½ cup almond milk
½ cup orange juice
2 tbsp lemon juice
1 tbsp honey or maple syrup
2 ice cubes

DIRECTIONS

1. Blend all the fixings in your blender until smooth.
2. Serve and enjoy!

Nutrition: Calories: 329; Fat: 17g; Carbs: 9g; Protein: 37g

Spiced Ginger Tea

 Prep Time: 10 minutes   Cooking Time: 5-10 minutes   Servings: 6

INGREDIENTS

8 cups water
1 (4-inch) piece of fresh ginger, chopped
4 lemons, sliced
6 cardamom pods, bruised
1 cinnamon stick
1 whole star anise pod
3 tbsp raw honey

DIRECTIONS

1. In a pan, add water over medium-high heat and bring to a boil. Stir in ginger, lemon slices, and spices, and adjust the heat to medium-low.
2. Simmer for 5-10 minutes and strain the tea into a pitcher. Stir in honey and serve.

Nutrition: Calories: 37; Fat: 0.1g; Carbs: 10.1g; Protein: 0.2g

---

Applesauce-Avocado Smoothie

 Prep Time: 5 minutes   Cooking Time: 0 minutes   Servings: 1

INGREDIENTS

1 cup unsweetened almond milk
½ avocado, pitted & sliced
½ cup applesauce
¼ tsp ground cinnamon
½ cup ice
½ tsp stevia or 1 tbsp honey for sweetness (optional)

DIRECTIONS

1. Blend all the fixings in your blender until smooth.
2. Serve and enjoy!

Nutrition: Calories: 270; Fat: 11g; Carbs: 4g; Protein: 39g

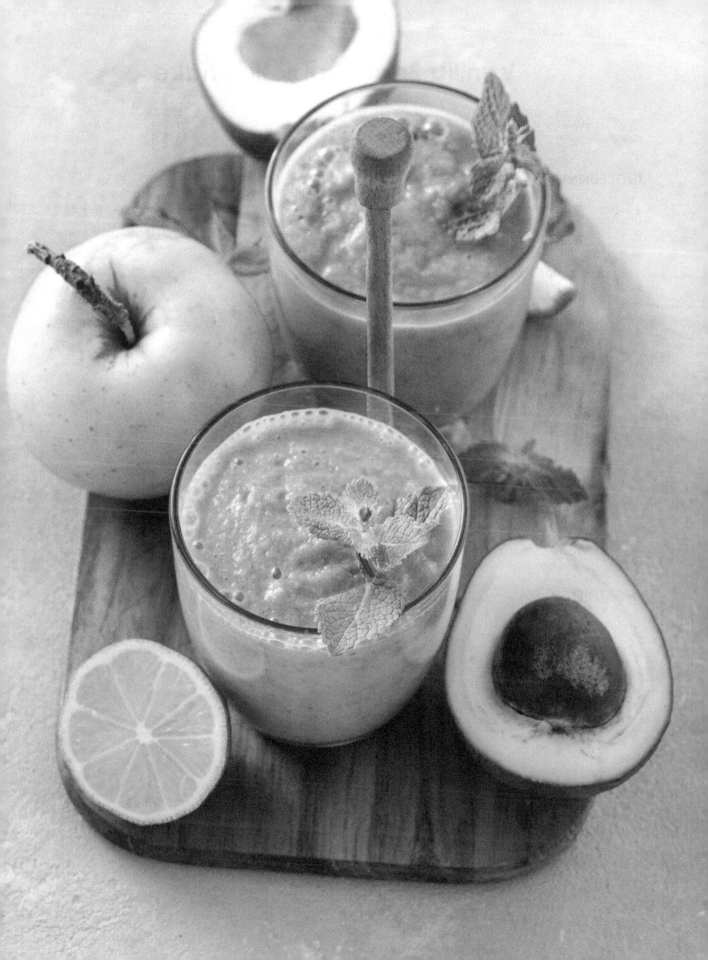

Vanilla Bean Probiotic Shake

 Prep Time: 5 minutes   Cooking Time: 0 minutes   Servings: 2

INGREDIENTS

1 cup low-fat milk or unsweetened vanilla soy milk
¼ cup low fat plain Greek yogurt
1 scoop (¼ cup) vanilla protein powder
½ cup low-fat plain kefir
5 ice cubes
1 tsp vanilla extract

DIRECTIONS

1. Combine yogurt, protein powder, kefir, ice cubes, vanilla, and milk in a blender.
2. Blend until powder is well dissolved for at least 3-4 minutes. Serve immediately.

Nutrition: Calories: 153; Carbs: 8g; Fat: 3g; Protein: 22g

Turmeric Lemon & Ginger Tea

 Prep Time: 10 minutes   Cooking Time: 10-12 minutes   Servings: 4

INGREDIENTS

6 cups water
½ of lemon, seeded & chopped roughly
1 (1-inch) piece of fresh ginger, chopped
2 tbsp maple syrup
¼ tsp ground turmeric

DIRECTIONS

1. In a saucepan, add all the ingredients over medium-high heat and bring to a boil.
2. Adjust the heat to medium-low and simmer for about 10-12 minutes. Strain into your cup and serve hot.

Nutrition: Calories: 32; Fat: 0.1g; Carbs: 8g; Protein: 0.2g

Sage Rosemary Tea

 Prep Time: 10 minutes + steeping time

 Cooking Time: 5 minutes

 Servings: 2

INGREDIENTS

2-3 cups of water
2 tbsp fresh sage leaves, crushed
1 tbsp fresh rosemary leaves, crushed

DIRECTIONS

1. Add the water to a saucepan and let it boil. Remove, cover and steep for 10 minutes.
2. Strain the tea and serve warm.

Nutrition: Calories: 2; Fat: 0.3g; Carbs: 1.4g; Protein: 0.3g

---

Cranberry Honey Juice

 Prep Time: 10 minutes

 Cooking Time: 0 minutes

 Servings: 4

INGREDIENTS

4 cups fresh cranberries
1 tbsp fresh lemon juice
2 cups of filtered water
1 tsp raw honey

DIRECTIONS

1. Put all the fixings in your blender and pulse until well combined.
2. Strain the juice through a cheesecloth-lined sieve and transfer it into four glasses. Serve immediately.

Nutrition: Calories: 66; Fat: 0g; Carbs: 11.5g; Protein: 0g

Carrot Orange Juice

 Prep Time: 10 minutes   Cooking Time: 0 minutes   Servings: 4

INGREDIENTS

2 pounds carrots,
trimmed & scrubbed
6 small oranges, peeled
& sectioned

DIRECTIONS

1. Add the carrots and orange sections into a juicer and extract the juice.
2. Through a cheesecloth-lined sieve, strain the juice and transfer it into four glasses. Serve immediately.

Nutrition: Calories: 130; Fat: 0.6g; Carbs: 31g; Protein: 2.2g

---

Refreshing Strawberry Smoothie

 Prep Time: 5 minutes   Cooking Time: 0 minutes   Servings: 1

INGREDIENTS

1 cup nonfat plain
Greek yogurt
1 cup frozen
unsweetened
strawberries
¼ tsp stevia

DIRECTIONS

1. Add the yogurt, strawberries, and stevia to a blender.
2. Blend on low within 2 minutes until completely combined. Enjoy immediately.

Nutrition: Calories: 170; Fat: 0g; Carbs: 20g; Protein: 24g

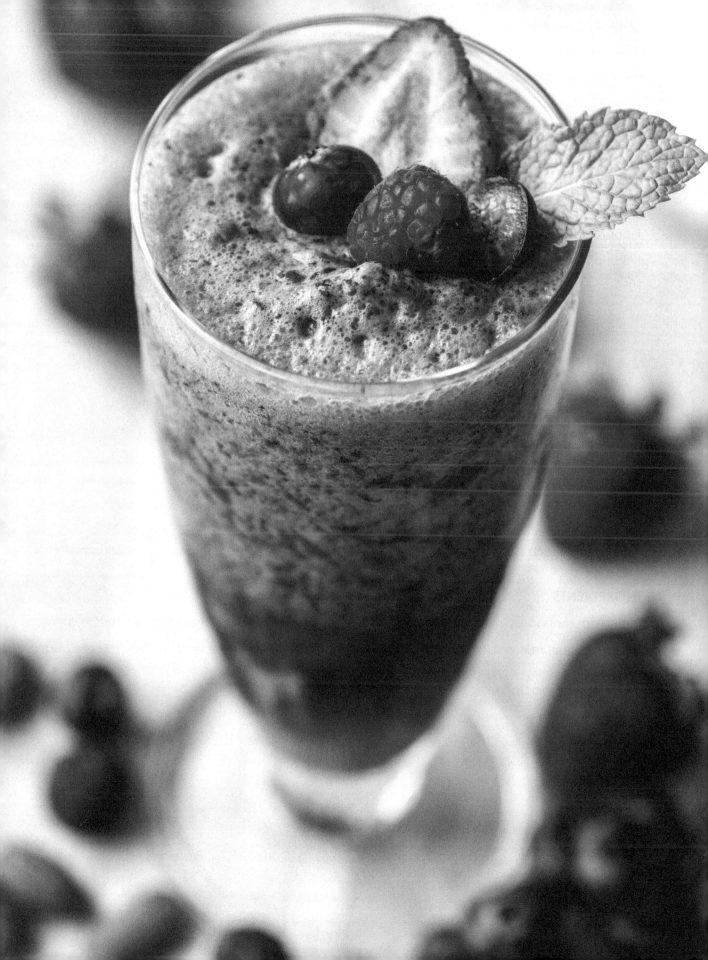

Apple-Cinnamon Tea

 Prep Time: 5 minutes   Cooking Time: 15 minutes   Servings: 4

INGREDIENTS

1 cup chopped apples
3 cinnamon sticks
1-quart water
2 bags of Earl Grey tea
1/3 cup honey, plus
more if desired

DIRECTIONS

1. Add the apples, cinnamon sticks, and water to a large saucepan over high heat. Bring to a boil. Set the heat to medium and stir for 15 minutes.
2. Remove from the heat and add the Earl Grey tea bags. Steep for 10 minutes.
3. Using a slotted spoon, detach the tea bags, apples, and cinnamon sticks. Attach the honey and stir until it dissolves. Taste and add more honey if desired. Serve hot.

Nutrition: Calories: 101; Fat: 1g; Carbs: 27g; Protein: 1g

Fresh Mango Smoothie

 Prep Time: 10 minutes   Cooking Time: 0 minutes   Servings: 3

INGREDIENTS

1 medium mango
roughly chopped
1 cup coconut milk
1 tbsp walnuts,
chopped.
1 tsp vanilla extract,
sugar-free

DIRECTIONS

1. Combine mango, coconut milk, walnuts, and vanilla extract in a blender and process until well combined and creamy.
2. Transfer to your serving glass and stir in the vanilla extract. Serve and enjoy.

Nutrition: Calories: 271; Fat: 21g; Carbs: 21.7g; Protein: 3.4g

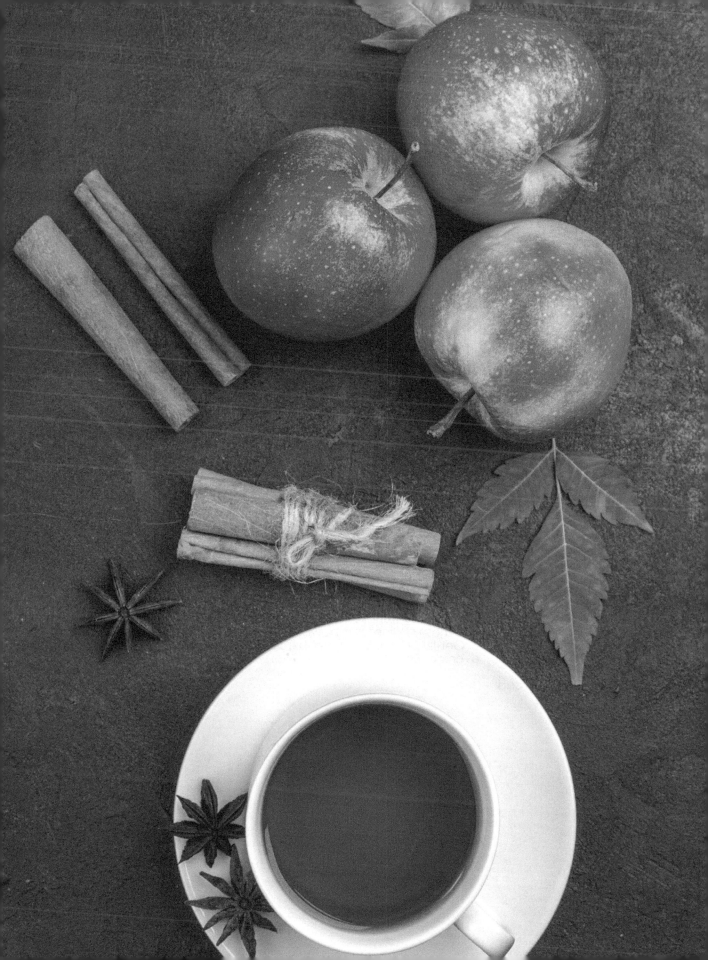

Citrus Green Tea

 Prep Time: 10 minutes   Cooking Time: 4 minutes   Servings: 4

INGREDIENTS

4 cups of filtered water
4 orange peel strips
4 lemon peel strips
4 green tea bags
2 tsp honey

DIRECTIONS

1. In a medium pan, add the water, orange, and lemon peel strips over medium-high heat and bring to a boil.
2. Set the heat to low and stir, uncovered, for about 10 minutes. With a slotted spoon, remove the orange and lemon peel strips and discard them.
3. Add the tea bags and turn off the heat. Immediately, cover the pan and steep for 3 minutes.
4. With a large spoon, gently press the tea bags against the pan to extract the tea completely. Remove the tea bags and discard them.
5. Add honey and stir until dissolved. Strain the tea in mugs and serve immediately.

Nutrition: Calories: 11; Fat: 0g; Carbs: 3g; Protein: 0g

Cucumber Cantaloupe Juice

 Prep Time: 10 minutes   Cooking Time: 0 minutes   Servings: 1

INGREDIENTS

1/4 lemon, peeled
2 stalks of celery
1/4 of a cantaloupe, peeled & cut into pieces
1/2 cucumber, sliced thinly

DIRECTIONS

1. Put all the fixings into your blender and pulse well. Strain the juice in a fine-mesh strainer in a bowl.
2. Gently press the pulp to extract all possible liquid, then discard it. Serve over ice. Enjoy!

Nutrition: Calories 69; Fat 0.2g; Carbs 13g; Protein 0.1g

Chilled Mint Green Tea

 Prep Time: 10 minutes   Cooking Time: 0 minutes   Servings: 2

INGREDIENTS

2 ½ cups boiling water
1 cup fresh mint leaves
4 green tea bags
2 tsp honey

DIRECTIONS

1. Mix the water, mint, and tea bags in a pitcher—cover and steep within 5 minutes.
2. Strain the tea mixture through a fine-mesh strainer into another pitcher. Refrigerate within 3 hours.
3. Discard the tea bags, then divide the tea in your serving glasses. Stir in honey and serve.

Nutrition: Calories: 41; Fat: 0.3g; Carbs: 9.6g; Protein: 1.5g

---

Celery Apple Juice

 Prep Time: 5 minutes   Cooking Time: 0 minutes   Servings: 2

INGREDIENTS

12 celery stalks, peeled & chopped
3 Apple, peeled, cored, seeded, & sliced
1-inch ginger root, peeled & chopped
1/4 lemon juice
2 cups water

DIRECTIONS

1. Put all the fixings into your blender and pulse well. Strain the juice in a fine-mesh strainer in a bowl.
2. Gently press the pulp to extract all possible liquid, then discard it. Serve over ice. Enjoy!

Nutrition: Calories: 116; Fat: 0.7g; Carbs: 28.2g; Protein: 1.5g

Orange Green Tea

 Prep Time: 10 minutes

 Cooking Time: 10 minutes

 Servings: 4

INGREDIENTS

4 cups of filtered water
6-8 orange peel strips
4 green tea bags
2 tsp honey

DIRECTIONS

1. In a medium pan, add the water, orange, and lemon peel strips over medium-high heat and bring to a boil.
2. Adjust the heat to low and simmer, uncovered, for about 10 minutes. With a slotted spoon, remove the orange and lemon peel strips and discard them.
3. Add in the tea bags and turn off the heat. Immediately cover the pan and steep for 3 minutes.
4. With a large spoon, gently press the tea bags against the pan to extract the tea completely. Remove the tea bags and discard them.
5. Add honey and stir until dissolved. Strain the tea in mugs and serve immediately.

Nutrition: Calories: 11; Fat: 0g; Carbs: 3g; Protein: 0g

Pineapple Mint Juice

 Prep Time: 5 minutes

 Cooking Time: 0 minutes

 Servings: 4

INGREDIENTS

3 cups pineapple, cored, sliced & chunks
10-12 mint leaves, or to taste
2 tbsp sugar, or to taste (optional)
1 ½ cup water
1 cup ice cubes

DIRECTIONS

1. Put all the fixings into your blender and pulse well. Strain the juice in a fine-mesh strainer in a bowl.
2. Gently press the pulp to extract all possible liquid, then discard it. Serve over ice. Enjoy!

Nutrition: Calories: 63; Fat: 1g; Carbs: 15.48g; Protein: 0.73g

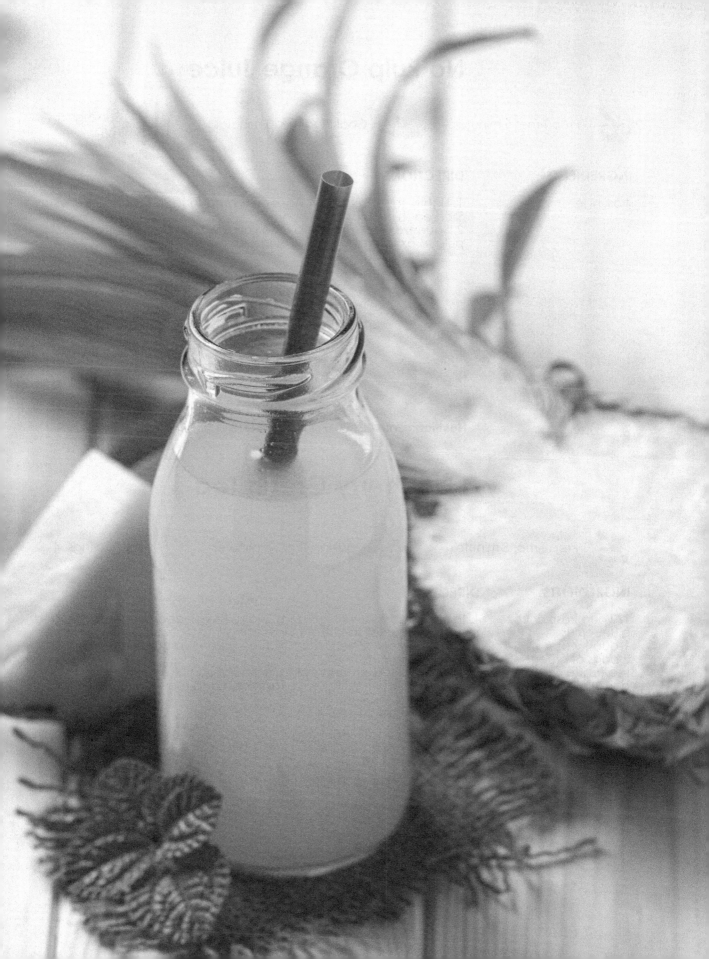

No Pulp Orange Juice

 Prep Time: 5 minutes

 Cooking Time: 0 minutes

 Servings: 1 ½ cup

INGREDIENTS

4 oranges

DIRECTIONS

1. Lightly squeeze the oranges on a hard surface to soften the exterior. Slice each in half.
2. Squeeze each orange over a fine-mesh strainer. Gently press the pulp to extract all possible liquid. Serve over ice. Enjoy!

Nutrition: Calories: 50; Fat: 0.2g; Carbs: 11.5g; Protein: 0.8g

---

Blueberry Green Tea

 Prep Time: 5 minutes

 Cooking Time: 5 minutes

 Servings: 4

INGREDIENTS

1/2 cup fresh or frozen blueberries
1-quart water
2 bags of green tea (caffeinated or decaffeinated)
1/3 cup honey, plus more if desired

DIRECTIONS

1. In a saucepan over high heat, place the blueberries and water and bring to a boil. Set the heat to low and stir for 5 minutes.
2. Detach from the heat and add the green tea bags. Steep for 10 minutes.
3. Using a slotted spoon, set the tea bags and blueberries. Attach the honey and stir until it dissolves. Taste and add more honey if desired. Serve hot.

Nutrition: Calories: 95; Fat: 0g; Carbs: 26g; Protein: 0.22g

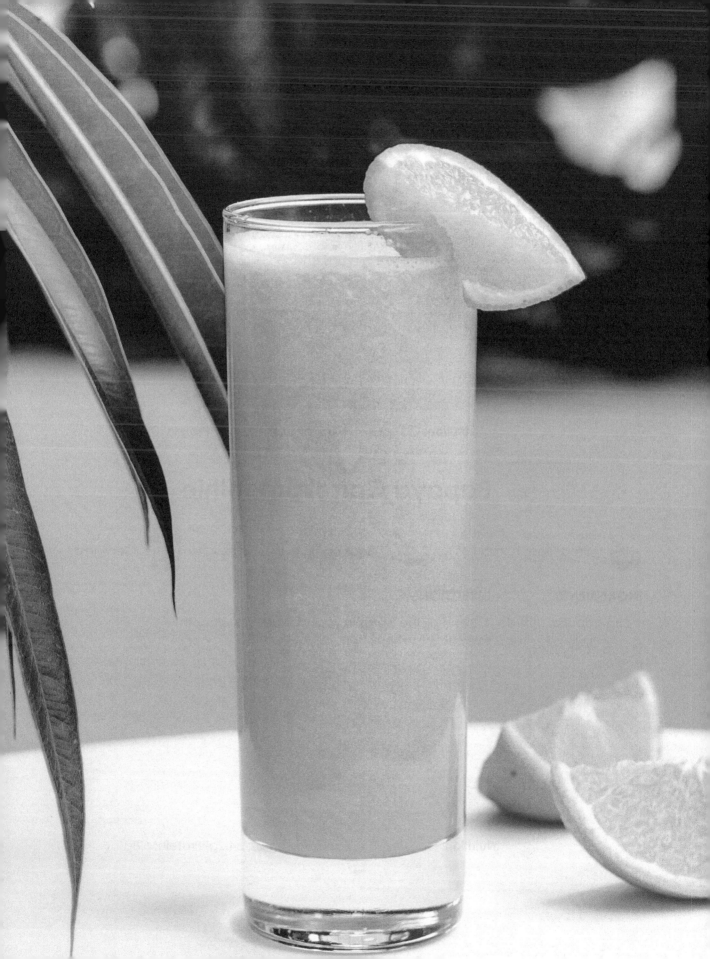

Lemony Black Tea

 Prep Time: 10 minutes   Cooking Time: 3 minutes   Servings: 6

INGREDIENTS

1 tbsp of black tea leaves
1 lemon, sliced thinly
1 cinnamon stick
6 cups boiling water

DIRECTIONS

1. Place the tea leaves, lemon slices, and cinnamon stick in a large teapot.
2. Pour hot water over the ingredients and immediately cover the teapot. Set aside for about 5 minutes to steep.
3. Strain the tea in mugs and serve immediately.

Nutrition: Calories: 4; Fat: 0g; Carbs: 0.82g; Protein: 0.1g

Papaya Carrot Smoothie

 Prep Time: 10 minutes   Cooking Time: 0 minutes   Servings: 1

INGREDIENTS

1 cup papaya, pitted
½ -¾ cup low-fat milk
½ cup canned carrot, peeled

DIRECTIONS

1. Blend all the fixings in your blender until smooth.
2. Serve and enjoy!

Nutrition: Calories: 186; Fat: 2.3g; Carbs: 34.2g; Protein: 6.8g

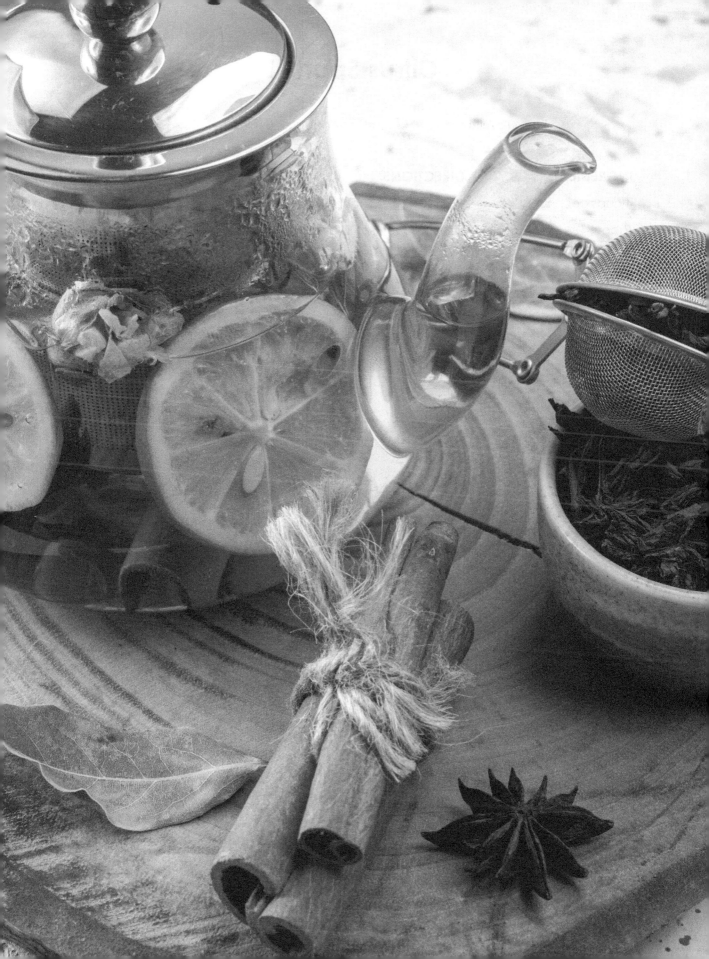

Citrus Sports Drink

 Prep Time: 10 minutes　　 Cooking Time: 0 minutes　　 Servings: 8

INGREDIENTS

4 cups coconut water
4 large oranges juice
(about 1 ½ cup),
strained
2 tbsp lemon juice,
strained
2 tbsp honey or maple
syrup
1 tsp sea salt

DIRECTIONS

1. Place the coconut water, orange juice, lemon juice, honey, and salt in a jug or pitcher.
2. Stir until the salt is dissolved, and serve cold.

Nutrition: Calories: 59; Fat: 1g; Carbs: 14g; Protein: 1g

Vanilla Apple Pie Shake

 Prep Time: 5 minutes　　 Cooking Time: 0 minutes　　 Servings: 2

INGREDIENTS

1 cup of low-fat milk
1 scoop (¼ cup)
vanilla protein
powder
1 small apple, peeled,
cored, and chopped.
1 tsp vanilla extract
2 tsp ground
cinnamon
½ tsp ground nutmeg
5 ice cubes

DIRECTIONS

1. Combine protein powder, apple, vanilla protein powder, cinnamon, nutmeg, ice cubes, and milk in a blender.
2. Blend until powder is well dissolved and no longer visible for at least 3-4 minutes. Serve immediately.

Nutrition: Calories: 123; Fat: 1g; Carbs: 14g; Protein: 14g

Apple Cider Water

 Prep Time: 5 minutes   Cooking Time: 0 minutes   Servings: 1

INGREDIENTS

8 oz water
1 tbsp apple cider vinegar
1 tbsp lemon juice
1 tsp maple syrup

DIRECTIONS

1. Add all the ingredients to a serving glass, and stir until maple syrup dissolves completely.
2. Serve immediately.

Nutrition: Calories: 24; Fat: 0.1g; Carbs: 4.9g; Protein: 0.1g

Lunch

Carrot Potato Soup

 Prep Time: 10 minutes   Cooking Time: 0 minutes   Servings: 2

INGREDIENTS

2 cups carrots, peeled & sliced
2 cups vegetable stock
1 cup potato, peeled & sliced
1 cup non-dairy milk
Himalayan salt to taste

DIRECTIONS

1. Add all the fixings to a saucepan and simmer for 25 minutes.
2. Blend using your immersion blender until smooth. Serve!

Nutrition: Calories: 174; Fat: 1.4g; Carbs: 28.6g; Protein: 6.5g

Creamy Shrimp Scampi

 Prep Time: 10 minutes   Cooking Time: 10 minutes   Servings: 1

INGREDIENTS

1 tbsp Greek yogurt, non-fat
1/2 minced garlic clove
4 shrimps
½ tbsp parsley chopped

DIRECTIONS

1. Add shrimps and 2 tbsp water to a hot pan, and cook for 2 to 3 minutes.
2. Add garlic and cook for 1 minute. Turn the heat off and add yogurt and parsley.
3. Puree using an immersion blender until smooth, and serve.

Nutrition: Calories 92, Protein 14 g, Carbs 0.9 g, Fat 3.7 g

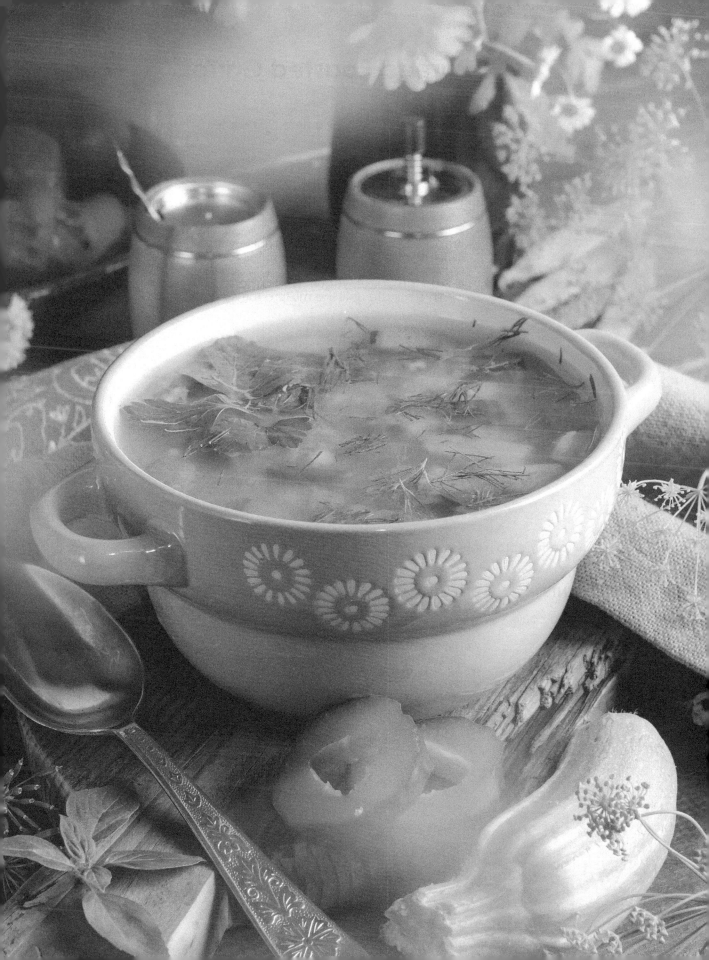

Pureed Roasted Carrot

 Prep Time: 5 minutes   Cooking Time: 30 minutes   Servings: 4

INGREDIENTS

1 cup peeled, sliced carrot
½ tbsp extra-virgin olive oil
Dash of salt
¾ cup non-fat plain Greek yogurt
¼ cup unsweetened almond milk

DIRECTIONS

1. Warm the oven to 425 F. Line a baking sheet with parchment paper and set aside.
2. In a bowl, toss the carrot and oil. Arrange the carrot slices on the prepared baking sheet and sprinkle with salt.
3. Bake within 25 to 30 minutes until the carrot softens and turns golden brown.
4. Add the carrot, yogurt, and almond milk to a blender. Blend on low within a minute until the mixture turns bright orange. Serve and enjoy.

Nutrition: Calories: 44; Fat: 2g; Carbs: 3g; Protein: 4g

Cauliflower Tofu Puree

 Prep Time: 15 minutes   Cooking Time: 45 minutes   Servings: 8

INGREDIENTS

1 large head cauliflower
Nonstick cooking spray
3 tbsp olive oil
¼ tsp salt
¼ tsp freshly ground black pepper
1 (8-oz) package soft tofu
1/3 cup low-sodium vegetable broth
1/8 tsp garlic powder

DIRECTIONS

1. Preheat the oven to 450°F.
2. Chop the cauliflower florets into even pieces. Spray a roasting pan with cooking spray and place the cauliflower in the pan.
3. Drizzle the oil on the florets, and sprinkle with salt and pepper. Toss, spread evenly, and cook in the oven for about 40 minutes.
4. Drain the tofu and press gently between paper towels to remove additional liquid.
5. In a food processor, combine the tofu, broth, garlic powder, and cooked cauliflower and blend well until smooth. Serve.

Nutrition: Calories: 159; Fat: 7g; Carbs: 7g; Protein: 20g

Pureed Turkey Tacos with Refried Beans

 Prep Time: 10 minutes   Cooking Time: 20 minutes   Servings: 1

INGREDIENTS

For the beans:

1/4 cup pinto beans, rinsed
1 tbsp chopped cilantro
¼ cup chicken broth, no-salt-added
¼ tsp minced garlic

For the turkey:

¼ cup ground turkey
1/8 tsp each of mild chili powder, cumin, garlic powder & paprika

DIRECTIONS

1.
2. Directions:
3. Sauté garlic in 2 tbsp of hot water for 1 minute, then add broth and beans.
4. Let it boil and simmer for five minutes. Mash with a masher, cook until liquid is gone, and mix with cilantro.
5. In a clean pan, sauté the turkey spices for 1 minute. Add turkey with 2 tbsp water and cook for 6 to 8 minutes. Add more water if needed.
6. Add the beans and turkey to the food processor, and pulse until smooth. Serve.

Nutrition: Calories 68, Protein 10.7 g, Carbs 0.5 g, Fat 0.9 g

---

Pureed Italian Chicken

 Prep Time: 10 minutes   Cooking Time: 1 minutes   Servings: 1

INGREDIENTS

1 tsp Italian seasoning
1 ½ tbsp tomato sauce
¼ cup canned chicken
salt & pepper, to taste

DIRECTIONS

1. Add the ingredients and puree with a stick blender in a bowl.
2. Microwave for 30 seconds, and serve.

Nutrition: Calories 106; Fat 4g; Carbs 3g; Protein 13g

Root Vegetable Soup

 Prep Time: 10 minutes   Cooking Time: 40 minutes   Servings: 1

INGREDIENTS

1 small sweet potato, peeled & cubed
5 cups water
1 leek, chopped
1 peeled parsnip, diced
1 chopped carrot
Salt & pepper to taste
1 turnip, peeled and diced
1/2 onion, diced

DIRECTIONS

1. In a large pan, add all ingredients. Stir and let it boil; simmer until all vegetables are tender. Drain all but 1 cup of water.
2. Puree with your immersion blender, and add more water to your desired consistency. Serve.

Nutrition: Calories 245; Fat 8.7g; Carbs 2.6g; Protein 18.2g

Creamy Carrot and Ginger Soup

 Prep Time: 10 minutes   Cooking Time: 30 minutes   Servings: 4

INGREDIENTS

1 tbsp coconut oil
1 chopped medium yellow onion
1 clove garlic minced
3 tbsp chopped fresh ginger
1 pound chopped and peeled carrots
24-32 oz vegetable broth
1 (14 oz) can of coconut cream
1/2 tsp salt + more as needed

DIRECTIONS

1. Heat your big skillet to medium-high heat. Dissolve the coconut oil in a saucepan over low heat.
2. Cook for about 5 minutes, or until the onion is soft and translucent, after which add the onion, garlic, and ginger.
3. Bring to a boil the carrots, vegetable broth, and stock.
4. Simmer the pot at a low temperature—Cook for 25 minutes, or until carrots are very soft. Add the coconut milk and whisk until mixed (or coconut cream if using).
5. Blend the soup until it's smooth using an immersion blender. Serve immediately.

Nutrition: Calories: 110; Fat: 3g; Carbs: 18g; Protein: 3g

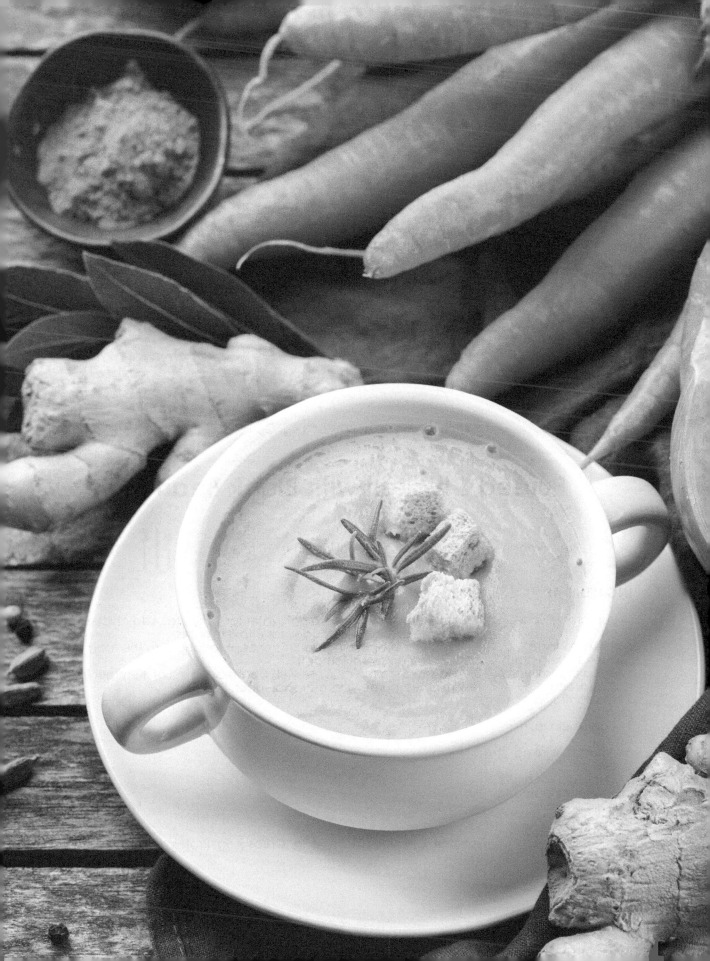

Pureed Ricotta & White Bean

 Prep Time: 10 minutes   Cooking Time: 5 minutes   Servings: 1

INGREDIENTS

2 tbsp chopped fresh parsley
¾ cup fat-free ricotta
¼ canned cannellini beans, with liquid
1/2 minced garlic clove

DIRECTIONS

1. In a pot, add beans with liquid and garlic. Let it boil, turn the heat low and simmer for 3 to 4 minutes.
2. Take it out in your bowl, and mix it with the rest of the ingredients—puree with a stick blender. Serve.

Nutrition: Calories 60; Fat 0.4g; Carbs 9.5g; Protein 4.7g

Pureed Chicken with Black Bean Mole

 Prep Time: 10 minutes   Cooking Time: 15 minutes   Servings: 2

INGREDIENTS

¼ cup ground chicken
paprika, to taste
¼ cup chicken broth
1/2 cup black beans: half cup, rinsed
1 tsp cilantro, chopped
1/2 garlic clove, minced
3 almonds, soaked overnight
1/8 tsp each of dried oregano, cinnamon, coriander, garlic powder
¼ tsp cacao powder

DIRECTIONS

1. Sauté the garlic in 1 tbsp hot water for 1 minute. Add chicken and more water, if necessary; cook for 6 to 8 minutes.
2. Add the rest of the ingredients except for beans to the food processor, and pulse until smooth.
3. Add sauce to the chicken with beans and stir. Let it simmer for a few minutes, puree with a stick blender. Serve.

Nutrition: Calories 109; Fat 3.9g; Carbs 9.5g; Protein 9.5g

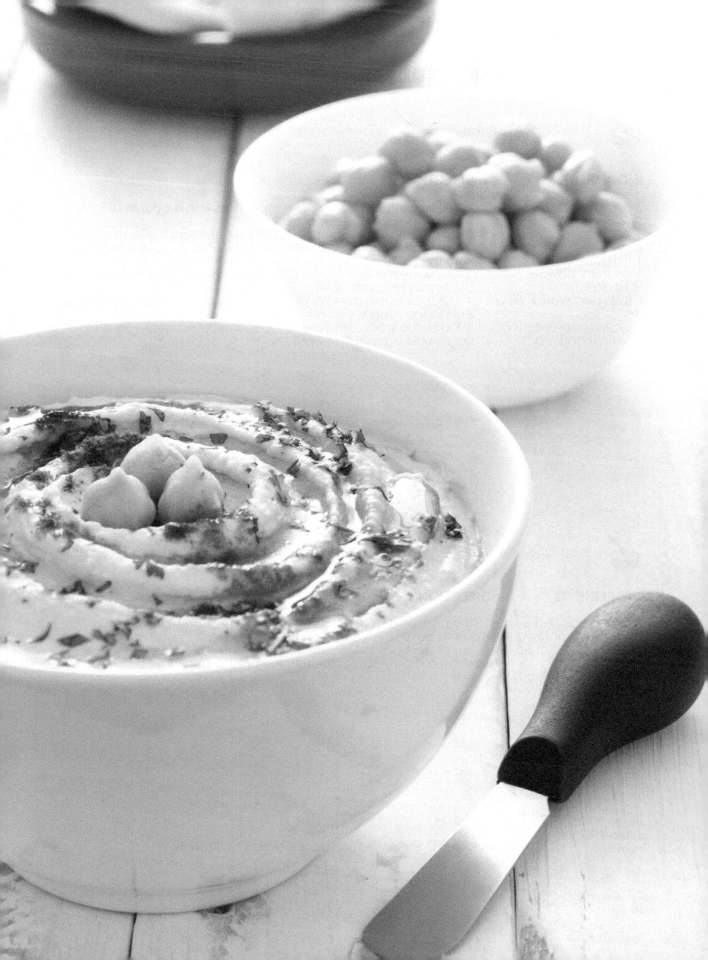

Butternut Squash Curry Soup

 Prep Time: 5 minutes   Cooking Time: 10 minutes   Servings: 4

INGREDIENTS

3 cups peeled and diced butternut squash
1 cup non-fat plain Greek yogurt
1 tsp garlic powder
1 tsp curry powder
½ tsp salt
2 tbsp pea protein powder
1½ cups unsweetened plain almond milk

DIRECTIONS

1. Fill the bottom of a medium saucepan with a couple of inches of water and insert a steamer basket.
2. Place the squash in the steamer basket, bring the water to a boil, and cover and steam for 7 to 8 minutes, until softened. Remove from the heat.
3. Combine the squash, yogurt, garlic powder, curry powder, and salt in your medium bowl.
4. Mix the protein powder plus almond milk in your separate small bowl. Add to the squash and mix well.
5. Place the mixture in your blender and blend on low for 30 to 60 seconds until smooth. Pour into bowls and enjoy.

Nutrition: Calories: 100; Fat: 2g; Carbs: 10g; Protein: 12g

Vegetable Broth

 Prep Time: 10 minutes   Cooking Time: 2-3 hours   Servings: 10

INGREDIENTS

4 carrots, peeled & chopped roughly
4 celery stalks, chopped roughly
3 parsnips, peeled & chopped roughly
2 large potatoes, peeled & chopped roughly
1 medium beet, trimmed & chopped roughly
1 large bunch of fresh parsley
1 (1 inch) fresh ginger, sliced
Filtered water, as needed

DIRECTIONS

1. In a pan, add all the ingredients over medium-high heat. Add enough water to cover the veggie mixture and bring to a boil.
2. Adjust the heat to low, cover, and simmer for about 2-3 hours. Through a fine-mesh sieve, strain the broth into a large bowl. Serve hot.

Nutrition: Calories: 76; Fat: 0.2g; Carbs: 17g; Protein: 2g

Pureed Lemon Garlic Salmon

 Prep Time: 10 minutes   Cooking Time: 0 minutes   Servings: 1

INGREDIENTS

¼ tsp garlic powder
1/6 tbsp mayonnaise, low-fat
2 oz canned salmon
1/3 tsp lemon juice

DIRECTIONS

1. Drain the salmon and transfer it to a food processor.
2. Add the rest of the ingredients, and pulse until smooth. Serve.

Nutrition: Calories 88; Fat 4g; Carbs 1g; Protein 11g

Red Lentil Mash

 Prep Time: 15 minutes   Cooking Time: 20 minutes   Servings: 8

INGREDIENTS

1 tbsp olive oil
4 garlic cloves, sliced
1 cup dry red lentils, rinsed
1 large carrot, chopped
½ tsp ground turmeric
½ tsp ground cumin
4 cups water
1 low-sodium vegetable bouillon cube

DIRECTIONS

1. In a large saucepan, heat the oil on medium-low heat. Add the garlic and stir until slightly brown, about 1 minute.
2. Add the lentils, carrot, turmeric, and cumin. Stir and cook to release the aroma, about 2 minutes.
3. Add the water and bouillon, then increase the heat to high and bring to a boil.
4. Once boiling, reduce the heat to low and simmer for about 20 minutes. The lentils will begin to fall apart when cooked.
5. Remove from the heat and let it cool. Divide into small batches and pulse in a blender to create a thick liquid. Strain to remove any pieces, and serve.

Nutrition: Calories 110; Fat 2g; Carbs 17g; Protein 6g

Pureed Buffalo Ranch Chicken

 Prep Time: 10 minutes   Cooking Time: 0 minutes   Servings: 1

INGREDIENTS

¼ cup sour cream, low-fat
1 canned chicken
4 oz cream cheese, low-fat
hot sauce, to taste
¼ packet of Mexican shredded cheese
1/2-packet ranch seasoning

DIRECTIONS

1. In a food processor, add all fixings and pulse until smooth
2. Serve and enjoy.

Nutrition: Calories 209; Fat 8.1g; Carbs 4.9g; Protein 21g

Egg Whites

 Prep Time: 10 minutes   Cooking Time: 10 minutes   Servings: 1

INGREDIENTS

2 egg whites
Salt & pepper to taste
Water, as needed

DIRECTIONS

1. Boil a pot of water. Swirl the water using your spoon, and add the egg whites to a large spoon.
2. Carefully add to the water. Cook until your egg white is no longer opaque, and take them out on a plate. Serve with salt and pepper.

Nutrition: Calories 56; Fat 1g; Carbs 1g; Protein 9g

Pureed Tuna-Avocado Salad

 Prep Time: 5 minutes   Cooking Time: 0 minutes   Servings: 1

INGREDIENTS

6 tbsp canned tuna,
drained
2 tbsp mashed avocado
2 tbsp diced red onion
Squeeze from 1 lemon
1/8 tsp dried cilantro
Salt (optional)
Freshly ground black
pepper (optional)

DIRECTIONS

1. Add the tuna, avocado, onion, lemon juice, and cilantro to a blender—season with salt (if using) and pepper (if using) to taste.
2. Blend on low within 1 minute or until completely combined. Serve and enjoy.

Nutrition: Calories: 113; Fat: 4g; Carbs: 5g; Protein: 17g

Lettuce Cucumber Soup

 Prep Time: 10 minutes   Cooking Time: 40 minutes   Servings: 2

INGREDIENTS

2 medium cucumbers, peeled, deseeded & diced
2 cups green lettuce, diced
3 cups vegetable stock
1 tbsp olive oil
1 tsp mustard powder
1 tsp basil dried
Himalayan salt, to taste

DIRECTIONS

1. Sauté the basil and mustard powder in your saucepan for 4-5 minutes over low heat.
2. Add the cucumbers and cook for 5 minutes. Add the stock and let it simmer for 30 minutes.
3. Transfer the mixture into a blender, add Himalayan salt to taste, and process until smooth. Serve warm.

Nutrition: Calories: 92; Fat: 7.2g; Carbs: 5.7g; Protein: 1.9g

Swede Soup

 Prep Time: 10 minutes   Cooking Time: 45 minutes   Servings: 6

INGREDIENTS

½ swede (rutabaga), peeled & cut into 12-inch cubes
2 parsnips, peeled & cut into 12-inch cubes
2 carrots, peeled & cut into 12-inch cubes
1 onion, peeled & cut into 12-inch cubes
2 tbsp olive oil
2 tsp ras el hanout
1 tsp oregano (dried)
3 cups stock (vegetable or chicken)
salt & pepper
To serve:
Fresh herbs (chopped)
drizzle cream or hemp or flax oil (or a knob of butter)

DIRECTIONS

1. Warm the oven to 400°F.
2. Put the vegetables in a roasting dish with a generous sprinkle of salt and oregano, then drizzle with olive oil. Stir to mix the oil and spices and ensure that the veggies are well-coated.
3. Roast in your oven within 15 minutes, remove and shake to mix well. Put it back into your oven and continue to roast within 15–25 minutes until the potatoes are tender.
4. In a large saucepan, mix the cooked veggies with the remaining ingredients. Save a few pieces for later use as a garnish if desired.
5. To get all the crispy bits from the bottom of the pan, use a spatula or wooden spoon to scrape the stock into the roasting dish.
6. Add the vegetable stock to the pot and heat through. Purée the soup with an immersion blender or a food processor.
7. Adjust the seasoning to your liking. Add a knob of butter to your soup for more richness and creaminess.
8. With just a squeeze of lemon juice, the flavors will be enlivened and made more vibrant.

Nutrition: Calories: 145, Fat: 1g; Carbs: 33g; Protein: 4g

Pureed Sweet Potato

 Prep Time: 10 minutes   Cooking Time: 5-6 minutes   Servings: 1

INGREDIENTS

1 tbsp butter
¼ tsp cinnamon
1/2 tsp salt
1 sweet potato
2 tbsp orange juice
¼ tsp nutmeg
1/2-packet stevia
black pepper, to taste
1 tbsp 0% milk

DIRECTIONS

1. Trim the potato and wrap it in parchment paper.
2. Microwave for 5 to 6 minutes. Cut the potato and transfer the soft flesh to a food processor.
3. Add the rest of the fixings, and pulse until smooth. Serve.

Nutrition: Calories 224; Fat 6g; Carbs 17.3g; Protein 7.3 g

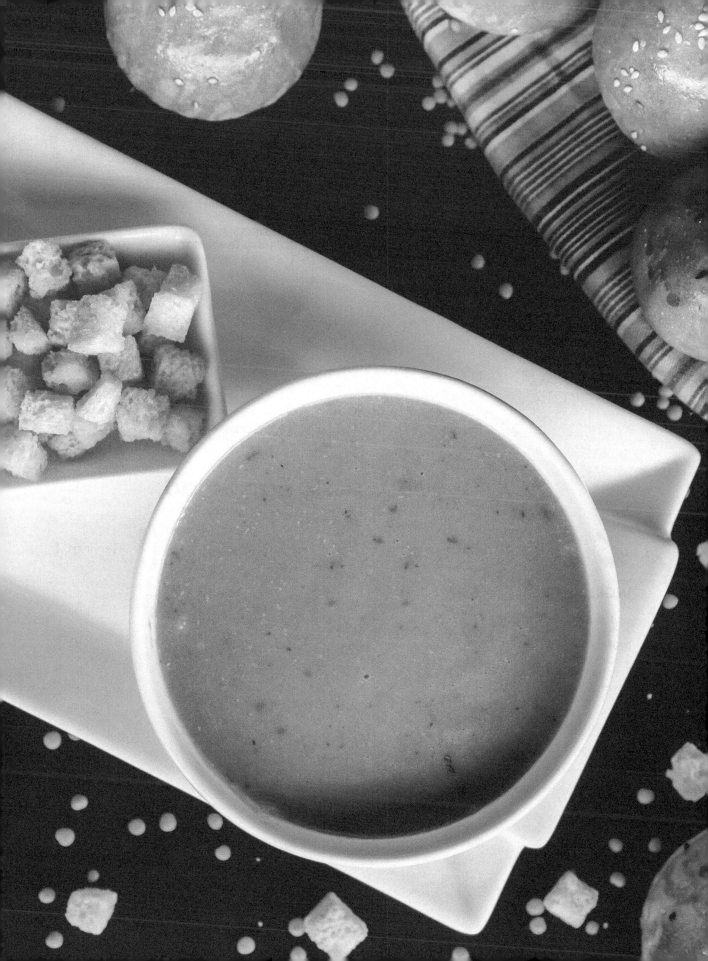

Chicken Carrot Broth

 Prep Time: 15 minutes

 Cooking Time: 2 hours & 5 minutes

 Servings: 8

INGREDIENTS

1 (3 pounds) chicken, cut into pieces
5 medium carrots
4 celery stalks with leaves
6 fresh thyme sprigs
Salt to taste
9 cups of cold water

DIRECTIONS

1. Add all the fixings to a large pan over medium-high heat and bring to a boil.
2. Set the heat to medium-low and stir, covered for about 2 hours, occasionally skimming the foam from the surface.
3. Strain the broth through your fine-mesh sieve into a large bowl. Serve hot.

Nutrition: Calories: 256; Fat: 16g; Carbs: 4.3g; Protein: 21.1g

---

Pureed Classic Egg Salad

 Prep Time: 10 minutes

 Cooking Time: 0 minutes

 Servings: 1

INGREDIENTS

salt & pepper to taste
1 tbsp mayonnaise, low-fat
1 soft-boiled egg
1 tbsp Greek yogurt, low-fat

DIRECTIONS

1. In a food processor, add all the ingredients.
2. Pulse until smooth, and serve!

Nutrition: Calories 176; Fat 13.2g; Carbs 4.6g; Protein 9.3g

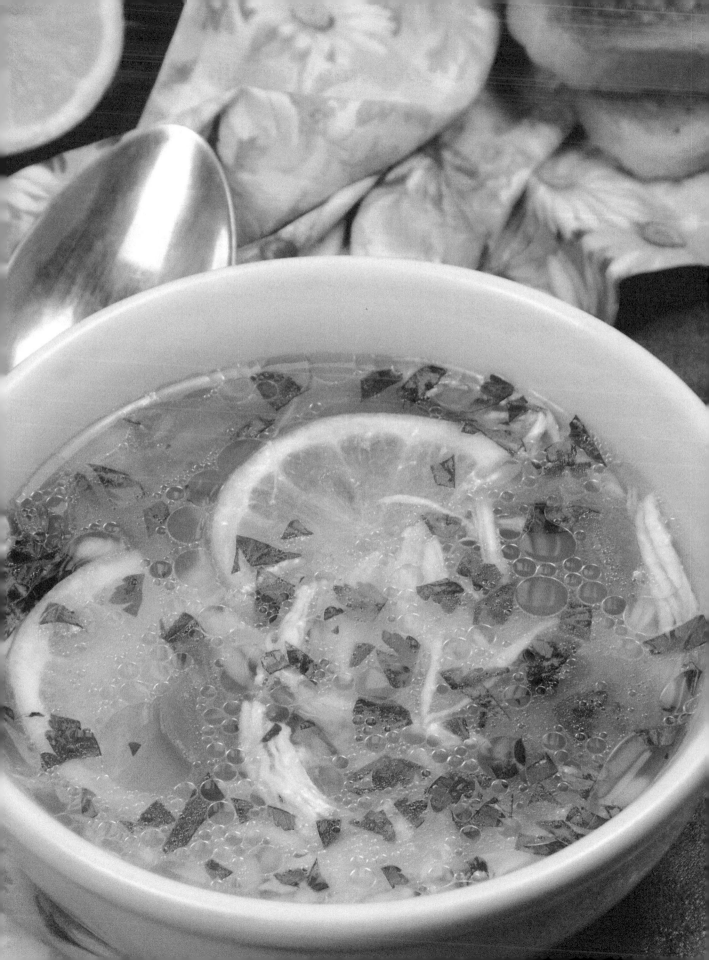

Clear Pumpkin Broth

 Prep Time: 15 minutes   Cooking Time: 30 minutes   Servings: 6

INGREDIENTS

6 cups water
2 tbsp ginger, minced
2 cups potatoes, peeled & diced
3 cups kabocha, peeled & diced
1 carrot, peeled and diced
1 onion, diced
1/2 cup scallions, chopped

DIRECTIONS

1. Transfer the bones and vegetables to your stockpot. Top with enough water to cover, then allow to come to a boil on high heat slowly.
2. Adjust to low heat and simmer for at least 30 minutes. Set and pour the mixture through a fine-mesh strainer into a large bowl. Taste and season with salt. Serve hot. Enjoy!

Nutrition: Calories: 71; Fat: 0.25g; Carbs: 16.1g; Protein: 1.84g

---

Pureed Refried Beans

 Prep Time: 10 minutes   Cooking Time: 7 minutes   Servings: 1

INGREDIENTS

1 tsp cilantro, chopped
¼ canned pinto beans, rinsed
1/6 tsp each of garlic powder, chili powder, cumin & onion powder
¼ cup vegetable broth

DIRECTIONS

1. Add the pinto beans with a splash of water and cook in a pan for 1 to 2 minutes. Add the rest of the fixings, and let it come to a boil. Cook until liquid is reduced by half.
2. Mash the beans to a desired pureed consistency. Serve.

Nutrition: Calories 85; Fat 0.8g; Carbs 14.3g; Protein 5.9g

Pumpkin Chicken Soup

 Prep Time: 15 minutes   Cooking Time: 30 minutes   Servings: 1

INGREDIENTS

1/6 cup chopped onion
1/2 tbsp minced garlic
1 tbsp low-fat heavy cream
1/6 cup diced celery
¼ tsp olive oil
1 tbsp fresh cilantro, chopped
1 cup chicken broth
1/6 cup diced carrots
1/2 cup chicken breast: half cup, shredded
salt & pepper, to taste
3 oz pumpkin puree

DIRECTIONS

1. In a pot, sauté all vegetables except for garlic in hot oil for 15 minutes, till vegetables are tender. Add garlic, and cook for 60 seconds.
2. Add the rest of the ingredients, puree with a stick blender. Serve.

Nutrition: Calories 275; Fat 3.9g; Carbs 3.8g; Protein 7.3g

Dinner

Pumpkin Carrot Soup

 Prep Time: 10 minutes   Cooking Time: 30 minutes   Servings: 2

INGREDIENTS

¼ tsp ground turmeric & curry powder
chili flakes, to taste
1 cup peeled & cubed carrots
salt & pepper, to taste
1 sliced garlic clove
1 tsp olive oil
1/3 cup coconut milk
1 cup peeled & cubed pumpkin
1/2 tsp lemon juice
1 ½ cups chicken broth, low-salt

DIRECTIONS

1. In a pot, sauté garlic in oil for 1 minute. Add spices and cook for 1 minute. Add vegetables and cook within a few minutes. Add the liquids, and let it come to a boil.
2. Turn the heat low and simmer within 15 minutes till the vegetables are tender. Turn the heat off, puree with a hand blender. Adjust seasoning and serve.

Nutrition: Calories 84; Fat 1g; Carbs 19g; Protein 3g

Pureed Ginger Garlic Tofu

 Prep Time: 10 minutes   Cooking Time: 10 minutes   Servings: 1

INGREDIENTS

4 oz firm tofu, cubed
¼ tsp minced ginger.
¼ tsp coconut aminos.
1/2 minced garlic clove

DIRECTIONS

1. Add all ingredients (except tofu) to a pan with ¼ cup of water.
2. Let it come to a boil, and add the tofu—Cook for 3 to 4 minutes. Add more water if needed—puree with a stick blender. Serve.

Nutrition: Calories 61; Fat 3.4g; Carbs 2.8g; Protein 6.9g

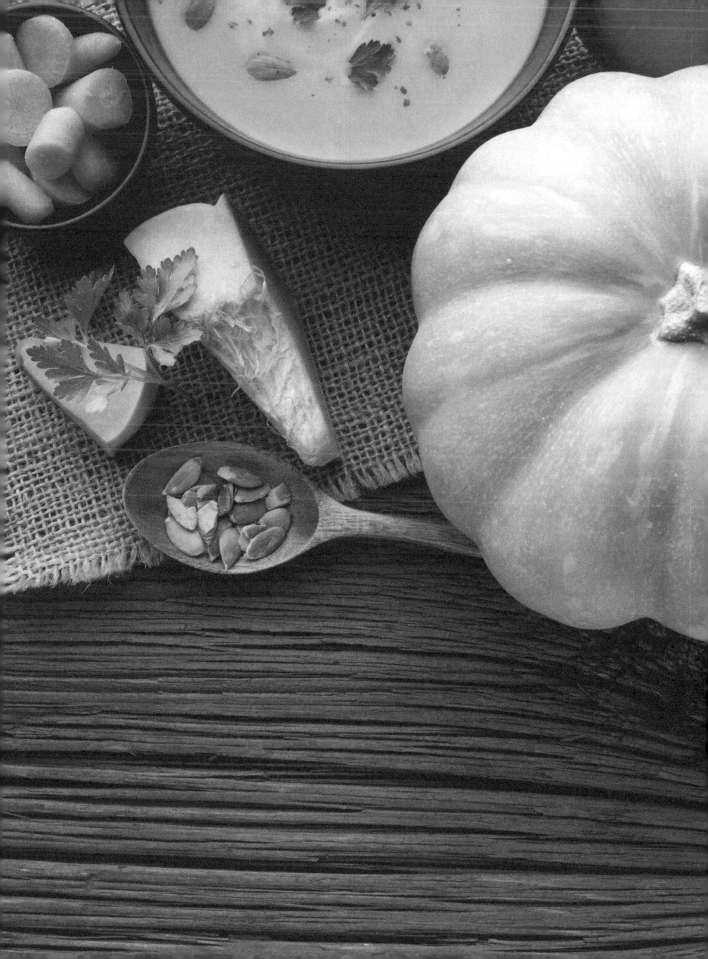

Pureed Moroccan Fish

 Prep Time: 10 minutes   Cooking Time: 10 minutes   Servings: 1

INGREDIENTS

1/2 clove of minced garlic
1/8 tsp each of paprika, cinnamon, turmeric & cumin
¼ cup coconut lite milk
¼ tsp apple cider vinegar
1 tbsp chopped fresh cilantro
4 oz white fish fillets
¼ cup canned chickpeas, rinsed

DIRECTIONS

1. In a pan, add dry spices and cook for 1 minute. Add garlic, vinegar, and 2 tbsp water, and cook for 1 to 2 minutes.
2. Add the rest of the ingredients, and cook on high. Let it boil, turn the heat low and simmer for 4 to 6 minutes.
3. Turn the heat off, and add cilantro. Puree with a stick blender, and serve!

Nutrition: Calories 67; Fat 1.2g; Carbs 6.8g; Protein 7g

Pureed Sesame Tuna Salad

 Prep Time: 10 minutes   Cooking Time: 0 minutes   Servings: 1

INGREDIENTS

¼ tsp tahini
1 tsp chopped parsley
¼ tsp apple cider vinegar
1/8 tsp coconut aminos
2 tbsp Greek yogurt, low-fat
¼ tsp sesame seeds
4 oz canned light tuna in water

DIRECTIONS

1. Whisk all ingredients except for fish.
2. Break the tuna and add to the mixture, puree, and serve.

Nutrition: Calories 78; Fat 3.4g; Carbs 1.3g; Protein 11.7g

Pureed Caribbean Pork

 Prep Time: 10 minutes   Cooking Time: 5 minutes   Servings: 1

INGREDIENTS

1/8 tsp dried thyme
1/8 tsp dried parsley
1 tsp chopped fresh cilantro
1/8 tsp allspice
1/8 tsp paprika
1/8 tsp garlic powder
1/4 tsp apple cider vinegar
1/2 cup ground pork
1/4 cup canned black beans

DIRECTIONS

1. In your pan, add all dry spices and herbs and cook for 1 minute. Add pork with 2 tbsp water on high heat. Cook for 4 to 5 minutes until done. Add more water if needed.
2. Add beans and vinegar, and cook for 1 to 2 minutes. Turn the heat off, and add cilantro. Pulse until smooth. Serve.

Nutrition: Calories 65; Fat 1.8g; Carbs 2.6g; Protein 9.8g

Pureed Rosemary Chicken with Blue Cheese

 Prep Time: 10 minutes   Cooking Time: 10 minutes   Servings: 1

INGREDIENTS

4 oz ground chicken
¼ cup canned chickpeas, rinsed
1/2 minced garlic clove
1/8 tsp toasted sunflower seeds, unsalted
1/4 tsp blue cheese, crumbled, low-fat
1/8 tsp apple cider vinegar
2 tbsp Greek yogurt low-fat
1 tsp fresh rosemary, chopped

DIRECTIONS

1. In a pan, add garlic with 2 tbsp water and cook for 1 minute. Add chicken and cook for 6 to 8 minutes. Add more water if your pan is dry.
2. Add chickpeas and rosemary, and cook for 2 to 3 minutes. Turn the heat off. Add the rest of the ingredients to a bowl and mix.
3. Transfer to the chicken mixture. Puree and serve.

Nutrition: Calories 135; Fat 2g; Carbs 3g; Protein 10.3g

Light Tomato Soup

 Prep Time: 10 minutes   Cooking Time: 20 minutes   Servings: 1

INGREDIENTS

1/2 onion, chopped
4 fresh tomatoes, chopped
1 minced clove of garlic
salt & pepper, to taste
¼ tsp olive oil
1 tbsp basil leaves, chopped
water, as needed

DIRECTIONS

1. Sauté the onion and garlic in hot oil. Add basil plus tomatoes, and cook until tender.
2. Add salt and pepper, puree with a stick blender. Add enough water and simmer for a few minutes, and serve.

Nutrition: Calories 144; Fat 5.9g; Carbs 6g; Protein 6.7g

Pureed Chili

 Prep Time: 10 minutes   Cooking Time: 40 minutes   Servings: 1

INGREDIENTS

¼ canned chili beans
1/4 green pepper
1/2 cup turkey meat
¼ canned diced tomatoes
¼ tsp ketchup
¼ canned pinto beans
2 tbsp tomato paste

DIRECTIONS

1. Add turkey plus green pepper to a pan, and cook until done. Add the rest of the fixings, and cook for 30-40 minutes.
2. Puree with a stick blender, serve, and enjoy.

Nutrition: Calories 267; Fat 12.9g; Carbs 12g; Protein 19.9g

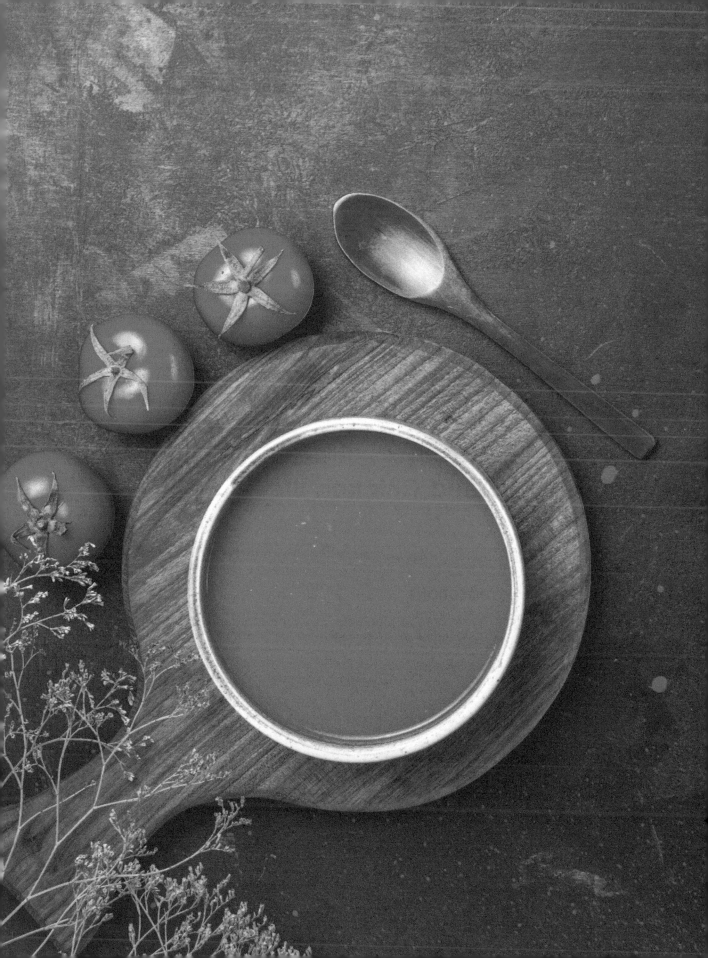

Pureed Mediterranean Chicken

 Prep Time: 10 minutes   Cooking Time: 10 minutes   Servings: 1

INGREDIENTS

¼ tsp tahini
1 tsp parsley, chopped
¼ tsp za'atar spice
3 oz ground chicken
¼ cup canned chickpeas, rinsed

DIRECTIONS

1. Add chicken and 2 tbsp water to a pan, and cook for 5 to 7 minutes on medium flame.
2. Add the rest of the ingredients to a bowl, mix and add to the chicken. Cook until heated through. Puree until smooth, serve.

Nutrition: Calories 89; Fat 4g; Carbs 2g, Protein 9g

Pureed Chicken Breast Salad

 Prep Time: 10 minutes   Cooking Time: 0 minutes   Servings: 1

INGREDIENTS

1 tbsp Greek yogurt, low-fat
salt & black pepper, as needed
1/2 chicken breast, cooked
1 tbsp mayonnaise, low-fat
1/8 tsp onion powder

DIRECTIONS

1. In your food processor, pulse the chicken until smooth.
2. Mix with the rest of the ingredients. Serve.

Nutrition: Calories 97; Fat 1.2g; Carbs 2.9g; Protein 14g

Creamy Cauliflower Soup

 Prep Time: 10 minutes   Cooking Time: 25 minutes   Servings: 3

INGREDIENTS

¼ cup raw cashews
2 tbsp olive oil
½ small white onion, diced
2 cloves garlic, minced
1 medium cauliflower, cut into 2-inch chunks
2 tbsp tahini (sesame paste)
salt and pepper to taste

DIRECTIONS

1. Soak the raw cashews covered in water for 8 hours or overnight, then drain well.
2. Heat oil in your Dutch oven over medium heat, and sauté onions and garlic until softened for about 5 minutes.
3. Pour 4 cups of water into your pot, chopped cauliflower, soaked and drained cashews, let it boil, reduce heat, then simmer until cauliflower fork-tender, about 15-20 minutes.
4. Remove soup from heat and let cool within 10 minutes. Stir in tahini. Transfer soup to your blender and puree until soup.
5. Season with salt plus pepper to taste and serve.

Nutrition: Calories: 146; Fat: 8g; Carbs: 10g; Protein: 7g

Pureed Cheeseburgers

 Prep Time: 10 minutes   Cooking Time: 20 minutes   Servings: 1

INGREDIENTS

1 minced garlic clove
¼ tsp olive oil
Worcestershire, to taste
1/2 cup ground meat of your choice
1 tbsp onion chopped
salt & pepper, to taste

DIRECTIONS

1. In a pan, sauté garlic and onion in hot oil. Add meat and cook until done; drain any oil.
2. Add the rest of the ingredients—Cook for a few minutes more. Puree with a stick blender, serve.

Nutrition: Calories 218; Fat 7g; Carbs 8g; Protein 20g

Beef Veggie Soup

 Prep Time: 10 minutes   Cooking Time: 35 minutes   Servings: 4

INGREDIENTS

1 tbsp extra-virgin olive oil
2 cups peeled, chopped carrot
1 cup chopped yellow onion
3 cups water
3 tsp powdered beef bouillon
1 tsp garlic powder
Nonstick cooking spray
8 oz lean ground beef

DIRECTIONS

1. In your medium pot, heat the oil over medium heat. Cook the carrot and onion for 5 to 7 minutes, frequently stirring, until the onion is translucent.
2. Add the water, bouillon, and garlic powder. Simmer within 5 minutes, occasionally stirring, to allow the flavors to develop.
3. While the broth simmers, heat a small skillet coated with nonstick cooking spray over medium heat. Place the beef in your skillet and cook for 5 minutes, or until the beef is no longer pink.
4. Remove from the heat and place the beef in the pot with the vegetables and broth.
5. Adjust the heat to medium-low, then simmer the soup for 20 minutes, or until the carrot has softened. Remove from heat and blend in your blender before serving.

Nutrition: Calories: 175; Fat: 8g; Carbs: 12g; Protein: 13g

Mexican Egg Puree

 Prep Time: 10 minutes   Cooking Time: 15 minutes   Servings: 1

INGREDIENTS

½ tbsp Greek yogurt, no-fat
2 tbsp canned black beans, rinsed
1/6 cup turkey sausage
1/8 tsp cumin
½ tbsp chopped cilantro
1 small egg
paprika, to taste

DIRECTIONS

1. Whisk egg with spices and yogurt—Cook sausage in a pan over medium flame for 5 to 6 minutes.
2. Add egg mixture and cook for 2 to 3 minutes. Add cilantro and beans, and cook for 1 minute.
3. Add 2 tablespoons of water and puree with a stick blender or a food processor. Serve.

Nutrition: Calories 128; Fat 7.1g; Carbs 2.6g; Protein 12.6g

Pureed Chicken & Sweet Potato

 Prep Time: 10 minutes   Cooking Time: 20 minutes   Servings: 1

INGREDIENTS

1/2 peeled sweet potato, cubed
½ Chicken breast, cooked

DIRECTIONS

1. In a pan, add sweet potato with water.
2. Cook for 10-15 minutes, until tender. Drain all but some liquid. Mash with a masher.
3. In your food processor, pulse the chicken until smooth. Add mashed sweet potato with the liquid.
4. Pulse until smooth. Adjust seasoning with salt and pepper. Serve.

Nutrition: Calories 45; Fat 1.9g; Carbs 3g; Protein 4g

Pureed Banana, Tofu & Pear

 Prep Time: 10 minutes   Cooking Time: 0 minutes   Servings: 1

INGREDIENTS

1/4 pear, peeled & chopped
2 oz tofu
1/2 banana

DIRECTIONS

1. In your food processor, add all fixings and pulse until smooth.
2. Serve and enjoy.

Nutrition: Calories 56; Fat 1g; Carbs 3.1g; Protein 4.9g

Pureed Cheesy Cauliflower

 Prep Time: 10 minutes   Cooking Time: 15 minutes   Servings: 1

INGREDIENTS

2 tbsp cream, low-fat
salt & pepper, to taste
1/2 tsp butter
1/2 cup cauliflower
florets
1 oz low-fat cheese

DIRECTIONS

1. In a bowl, add florets with butter and cream. Microwave for 4-6 minutes.
2. Mix and microwave for 4-6 minutes more—pulse in a food processor with cheese. Adjust seasoning and serve.

Nutrition: Calories 146; Fat 11g; Carbs 4g; Protein 6g

Mushroom Veggie Soup

 Prep Time: 10 minutes   Cooking Time: 35-40 minutes   Servings: 2

INGREDIENTS

1 zucchini, peeled,
seeded & diced
3 cups water
2 ½ cups vegetable
stock
2 cups mushroom,
chopped
1 cup beet, peeled &
shredded
1 cup lettuce, chopped
1 stalk of parsley,
chopped
1 tsp dried oregano
1 tsp olive oil
Himalayan salt, to
taste

DIRECTIONS

1. Cook the vegetables in a large saucepan with olive oil for a few minutes. Add the parsley and oregano, then cook for 6-10 minutes.
2. Add the vegetable stock and let it boil. Adjust to a simmer, and cook for 25 minutes. Blend using your immersion blender until smooth. Serve!

Nutrition: Calories: 87; Fat: 3.1g; Carbs: 12.1g; Protein: 5.5g

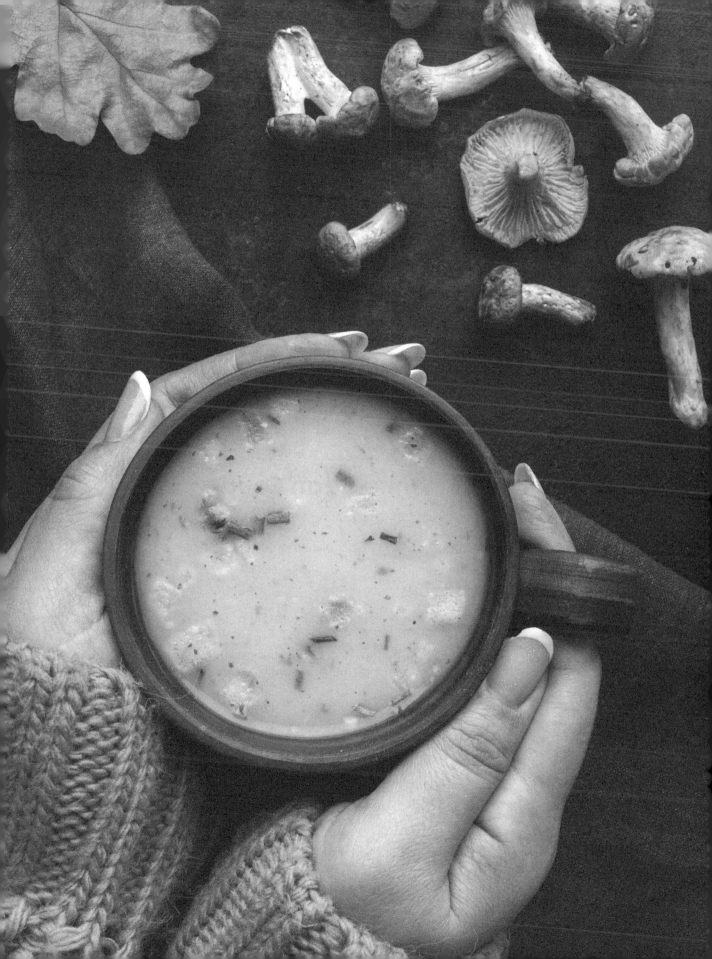

Pureed Chimichurri Chicken

 Prep Time: 10 minutes   Cooking Time: 15 minutes   Servings: 1

INGREDIENTS

1/8 tsp paprika
¼ cup ground chicken
2 tbsp chopped parsley
¼ tsp apple cider vinegar
1 tbsp cilantro
1/8 tsp dried oregano
1 clove of garlic

DIRECTIONS

1. Add two tablespoons of water and heat in a pan on medium flame. Add chicken, oregano, and paprika; cook for 6 to 8 minutes. Add more water if necessary.
2. Add the rest of the ingredients to a food processor, and pulse until smooth. Add the chimichurri to the chicken. Toss well and pulse in the food processor. Serve.

Nutrition: Calories 47; Fat 2.3g; Carbs 0.5g; Protein 5.6g

White Bean Soup

 Prep Time: 10 minutes   Cooking Time: 30 minutes   Servings: 1

INGREDIENTS

1/2 carrots, chopped
¼ tsp oregano
1/4 onion, chopped
1/2 minced garlic cloves, minced
1/8 tsp paprika
1 cup chicken broth, no-salt-added
1/2 cup green beans
1/2 celery sticks, chopped
¼ tsp tomato paste
¼ canned white beans
salt & pepper, to taste
¼ canned tomatoes
1/2 bay leaf

DIRECTIONS

1. Sauté celery, onion, and carrots in a splash of water for 10 minutes. Add paprika, garlic, and oregano, and cook for 45 to 60 seconds.
2. Add the rest of the fixings, stir well and let it come to a boil. Turn the heat low and simmer for 20 minutes, covered.
3. Adjust seasoning and puree with a stick blender. Serve.

Nutrition: Calories 191; Fat 4g; Carbs 33g; Protein 9g

Pureed Butternut Squash

 Prep Time: 5 minutes   Cooking Time: 15 minutes   Servings: 4

INGREDIENTS

2 cups diced butternut squash
1 cup nonfat plain Greek yogurt
½ cup shredded Parmesan cheese
½ tsp garlic powder
¼ tsp dried sage
¼ tsp salt

DIRECTIONS

1. Fill the bottom of your medium saucepan with a couple of inches of water and insert a steamer basket.
2. Place the squash in your steamer basket and bring the water to a boil—cover and steam for 15 minutes or until soft. Remove from the heat.
3. Add the butternut squash, yogurt, Parmesan cheese, garlic powder, sage, and salt to a blender or food processor. Blend the mixture for about 2 minutes or until smooth. Enjoy.

Nutrition: Calories: 104; Fat: 3g; Carbs: 11g; Protein: 11g

Lettuce And Spinach Soup

 Prep Time: 10 minutes   Cooking Time: 35 minutes   Servings: 2

INGREDIENTS

2 cups spinach fresh, chopped (if tolerated)
1 cup lettuce
3 cups vegetable stock
2 tsp olive oil
1 tsp cilantro
1 tsp whey protein
Himalayan salt to taste

DIRECTIONS

1. Sauté the veggies in a large saucepan for 5 minutes. Add the remaining fixings, and let it boil.
2. Adjust to a simmer, and cook for about 30 minutes. Blend using your immersion blender until smooth, and serve!

Nutrition: Calories: 61; Fat: 4.7g; Carbs: 1.9g; Protein: 3.6g

Ground Pork Sloppy Joe

 Prep Time: 5 minutes   Cooking Time: 10 minutes   Servings: 4

INGREDIENTS

1 tbsp extra-virgin olive oil
8 ounces lean ground pork
1 cup chopped yellow onion
1 cup canned diced tomatoes, drained
1 tbsp apple cider vinegar
1 tbsp brown sugar
1 tsp salt

DIRECTIONS

1. In your large skillet, heat the oil over medium heat. Cook the pork and onion for 7 to 9 minutes, frequently stirring, until cooked through.
2. Remove the skillet and drain the fat from the pork.
3. Return the skillet to the heat and add the tomatoes, apple cider vinegar, brown sugar, and salt.
4. Adjust the heat to medium-low then simmer within 2 minutes. Blend in your blender before serving.

Nutrition: Calories: 172; Fat: 9g; Carbs: 10g; Protein: 13g

Beef and Butternut Squash Stew

 Prep Time: 10 minutes   Cooking Time: 35 minutes   Servings: 4

INGREDIENTS

1 tbsp extra-virgin olive oil
1½ cups cubed butternut squash
1 cup chopped yellow onion
3 cups water
2 tbsp cornstarch
3 tsp powdered beef bouillon
1 tsp garlic powder
Nonstick cooking spray
12 ounces lean ground beef

DIRECTIONS

1. In your medium pot, heat the oil over medium heat. Cook the butternut squash and onion for 5 to 7 minutes, frequently stirring, until the onion is translucent.
2. Mix the water plus cornstarch to make a slurry in a small bowl. Add the slurry to the pot, stirring while pouring to ensure you transfer as much cornstarch as possible to the soup.
3. Add the bouillon and garlic powder. Simmer for about 5 minutes, stirring occasionally.
4. While the broth simmers, coat a small skillet with nonstick cooking spray and heat over medium heat.
5. Place the beef in the skillet and cook for 5 minutes, or until the beef is no longer pink. Remove from the heat and place the beef in the pot.
6. Reduce the heat to medium-low and simmer the soup for about 20 minutes, or until the squash has softened and the broth has thickened.
7. Remove from the heat and puree using an immersion blender until smooth before serving.

Nutrition: Calories: 237; Fat: 10g; Carbs: 18g; Protein: 19g

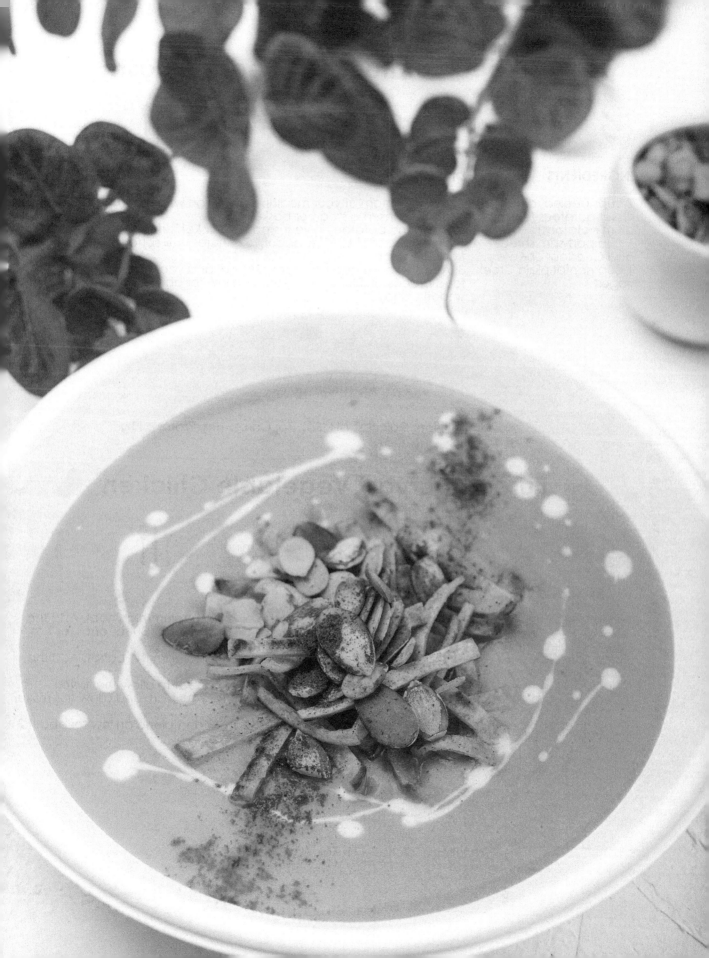

Pureed Potato and Cheddar Mash

 Prep Time: 10 minutes   Cooking Time: 15 minutes   Servings: 5

INGREDIENTS

2 cups peeled, diced russet potatoes (2½ medium potatoes)
1 cup part-skim shredded Cheddar cheese
1 cup nonfat plain Greek yogurt

DIRECTIONS

1. Fill the bottom of your medium saucepan with a couple of inches of water and insert a steamer basket.
2. Place the potatoes in your steamer basket, bring the water to a boil, and cover and steam for about 15 minutes until softened. Remove from the heat.
3. Add the potatoes, Cheddar cheese, and yogurt to a blender or food processor. Blend the mixture on low for about 2 minutes or until smooth. Enjoy.

Nutrition: Calories: 144; Fat: 7g; Carbs: 10g; Protein: 11g

Pureed Harvest Vegetable Chicken

 Prep Time: 10 minutes   Cooking Time: 25 minutes   Servings: 4

INGREDIENTS

1 tbsp extra-virgin olive oil
2 cups peeled, thinly sliced carrot
½ cup diced yellow onion
1 cup shredded chicken breast
1 cup chicken broth
¼ tsp salt

DIRECTIONS

1. In your large saucepan, heat the oil over medium-high heat. Add the carrot and onion to the pan and cook, stirring every 30 seconds for 7 to 9 minutes.
2. Pour a few tbsp of water if needed to help steam the carrot. Add the chicken, broth, and salt to the pan.
3. Simmer for another 7 to 9 minutes on low heat to allow the flavors to develop. Turn off the heat, then remove your pan, and allow the mixture to cool for 5 to 7 minutes.
4. Place the cooled mixture in your blender and blend on low for about 2 minutes or until smooth. Enjoy.

Nutrition: Calories: 171; Fat: 6g; Carbs: 6g; Protein: 19g

Snacks and Desserts

 Prep Time: 10 minutes + chilling time

 Cooking Time: 3 minutes

 Servings: 4

INGREDIENTS

8 large oranges juice (about 3 cups), strained & divided
2 tbsp unflavored gelatin
2 tbsp honey or maple syrup

DIRECTIONS

1. In a large bowl, pour 1/2 cup of orange juice and sprinkle with gelatin. Whisk well and let sit until the gelatin begins to set but is not relatively smooth.
2. In a saucepan over low heat, pour in the remaining 2 ½ cups of orange juice and cook until just before boiling, 2-3 minutes.
3. Remove and pour the hot juice into the gelatin mixture. Mix in the honey or maple syrup until the gelatin is dissolved.
4. Pour into an 8 x 8 inches baking dish and transfer to the refrigerator. Cool for 4 hours to set. Serve cold.

Nutrition: Calories: 153; Fat: 1g; Carbs: 27.4g; Protein: 9.76g

Strawberry Peach Pops

 Prep Time: 10 minutes + freezing time

 Cooking Time: 10 minutes

 Servings: 5

INGREDIENTS

1/2 cup stevia
6 oz canned strawberries
6 oz canned peaches
4 oz water
1 tbsp lemon juice

DIRECTIONS

1. Boil the water and stevia in your saucepan over medium heat. Allow the mixture to simmer, stirring until the sugar dissolves. Let it cool.
2. Add all the fixings into your blender, and blend until smooth. Set a fine-mesh strainer in a bowl, and strain the juice.
3. Pour your juice into your ice-pop molds, filling every three-quarters of the way. Add in your ice pop sticks, then set to freeze for at least 5 hours or until solid. Serve!

Nutrition: Calories: 99; Fat: 0.1g; Carbs: 25g; Protein: 0.4g

Cranberry-Kombucha Jell-O

 Prep Time: 5 minutes   Cooking Time: 0 minutes   Servings: 6

INGREDIENTS

1/4 cup room tempera-
ture water
1/4 cup hot water
1 tbsp gelatin
1 cup cranberry kombu-
cha, unsweetened

DIRECTIONS

1. Combine your gelatin and room temperature water, stirring until fully dissolved. Stir in hot water, then leave to rest for about 2 minutes.
2. Add in the kombucha and stir until combined. Transfer to serving-size containers, then place on a tray in the refrigerator to set for about 4 hours. Serve!

Nutrition: Calories: 13; Fat: 0g; Carbs: 2.1g; Protein: 1g

Orange Sugar-Free Gelatin

 Prep Time: 10 minutes   Cooking Time: 0 minutes   Servings: 6-8

INGREDIENTS

1/4 cup room tempe-
rature water
1/4 cup hot water
1 tbsp gelatin
1 cup orange juice,
unsweetened

DIRECTIONS

1. Combine your gelatin and room temperature water, stirring until fully dissolved. Stir in hot water, then leave to rest for about 2 minutes.
2. Add in the juice and stir until combined. Transfer to serving-size containers, then place on a tray in the refrigerator to set for about 4 hours. Serve!

Nutrition: Calories: 17; Fat: 0g; Carbs: 3.2g; Protein: 0.9g

Pumpkin Fluff

 Prep Time: 10 minutes + chilling time

 Cooking Time: 0 minutes

 Servings: 4

INGREDIENTS

1 (15 oz.) can of pumpkin puree
1 tsp pumpkin pie spice
1 cup skim milk
1 cup fat-free Cool Whip
1 small package of sugar-free vanilla pudding mix

DIRECTIONS

1. Mix the milk, pumpkin, and spice until well blended in a small bowl. Add the pudding mix and beat for 2 minutes.
2. Add the cold whip and refrigerate. Serve cold.

Nutrition: Calories: 79; Fat: 2g; Carbs: 15g; Protein: 1g

Honey Lemonade Popsicles

 Prep Time: 10 minutes + freezing time

 Cooking Time: 0 minutes

 Servings: 2

INGREDIENTS

1/2 cup honey
12 oz lemon juice
6 oz water

DIRECTIONS

1. Mix the honey and water in your saucepan over medium heat. Allow the mixture to simmer, stirring until the honey melts. Let it cool.
2. In a spouted container, combine all your ingredients. Pour your juice into your ice-pop molds, filling every three-quarters of the way.
3. Add in your ice pop sticks, then set to freeze for at least 5 hours or until solid. Serve.

Nutrition: Calories: 292; Fat:0.4g; Carbs: 30.9g; Protein: 0.8g

Strawberry Lemon Jell-O

 Prep Time: 10 minutes   Cooking Time: 0 minutes   Servings: 4

INGREDIENTS

2 scoops or 2 packets of strawberry sorbet
1 package Jell-O sugar-free lemon gelatin
2 cups water

DIRECTIONS

1. Dissolve the Jell-O in 1 cup of boiling water. After dissolving, set aside to cool for 3 to 5 minutes.
2. In your different bowl, measure 1 cup of cold water. Add two scoops or packets of Strawberry Sorbet to cold water, one scoop or packet at a time, stirring slowly to dissolve.
3. Stir sorbet mix in cold water with dissolved Jell-O. Cool quickly, and serve!

Nutrition: Calories: 60; Fat: 0g; Carbs: 2g; Protein: 12g

Low Fat Panna Cotta

 Prep Time: 10 minutes   Cooking Time: 5 minutes   Servings: 4

INGREDIENTS

½ tbsp gelatin
1 tbsp water
1 cup skim milk
2 tbsp pure maple syrup
1 cup low-fat buttermilk
1 cup low-fat Greek yogurt

DIRECTIONS

1. Mix the gelatin with the water in your small bowl and let stand until softened, about 5 minutes.
2. Bring the milk to a simmer with the maple syrup in a small saucepan. Remove from the heat and stir in the softened gelatin until it is dissolved.
3. Whisk the buttermilk with the yogurt in a medium bowl. Drizzle in the warm milk and whisk continuously until the panna cotta mixture is smooth.
4. Pour the panna cotta mixture into six 4-ounce ramekins, and refrigerate until set, about 3 hours.

Nutrition: Calories: 111; Fat: 1g; Carbs: 19g; Protein: 8g

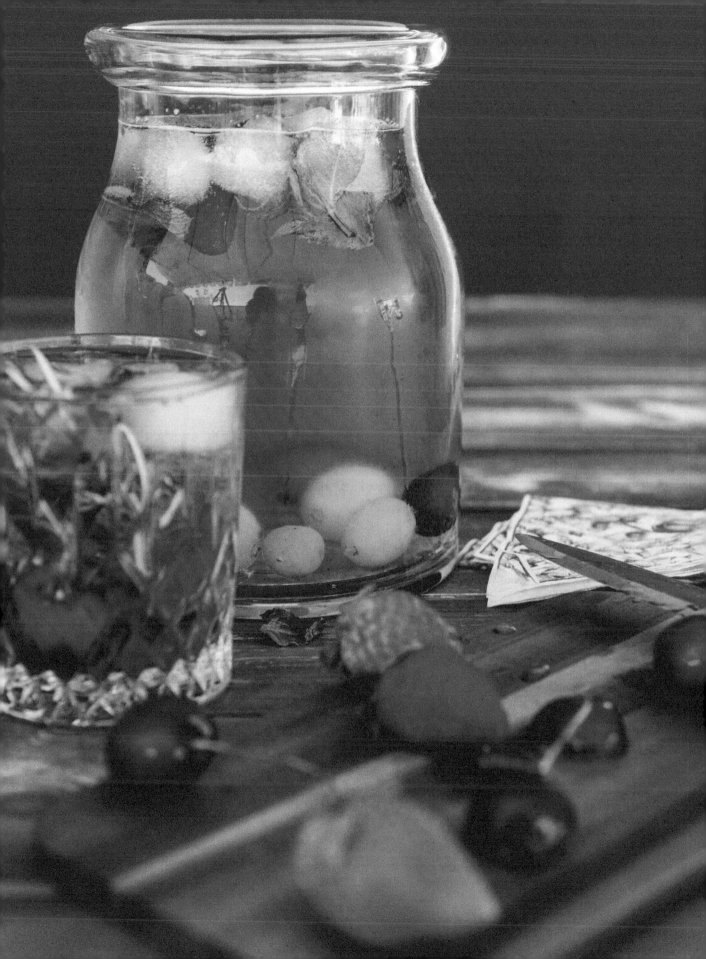

Easy Egg Custard

 Prep Time: 10 minutes

 Cooking Time: 20 minutes

 Servings: 1

INGREDIENTS

1/4 cup granulated sugar substitute
1 tsp cornstarch
¾ cup skim milk
1/4 tsp vanilla extract
1 egg yolk

DIRECTIONS

1. In a pan, add sugar, extract, and milk. Place on low flame, do not boil or simmer but make sure sugar dissolves. Whisk well the egg yolks with cornstarch
2. Turn the flame off and add a few tablespoons of warm milk to the egg mixture. Mix well and pour half of the warm milk mixture while keep whisking.
3. Add the rest and pour the mixture back into the pan—place on low flame, whisking until it thickens. Serve warm.

Nutrition: Calories 209; Carbs 33g; Fat 5.8g; Protein 6g

Blackberry-Rose Ice Pops

 Prep Time: 10 minutes + chilling time

 Cooking Time: 10 minutes

 Servings: 10

INGREDIENTS

5 cups blackberries
3 cups coconut water
1 tsp rosewater
1 tbsp lemon juice
9 tbsp cane sugar
9 tbsp water

DIRECTIONS

1. Mix the sugar plus water in a pan over medium heat until dissolved. Add the rest of the ingredients to a blender and pulse until smooth.
2. Pour the mixture and sugar syrup through a fine-mesh strainer into a large bowl. Pour in the molds and keep in the freezer until they are set. Serve.

Nutrition: Calories 45; Fat 5.3g; Carbs 11g; Protein 0.8g

Peach Gelatin

 Prep Time: 10 minutes   Cooking Time: 5 minutes   Servings: 10

INGREDIENTS

2 tbsp grass-fed gelatin powder
4 cups fresh peach juice, divided
2 tbsp honey

DIRECTIONS

1. In a bowl, soak the gelatin in ½ cup of juice and set aside for about 5 minutes.
2. In a medium pan, add the remaining juice over medium heat and bring to a gentle boil. Remove and stir in honey.
3. Pour the gelatin mixture and stir until dissolved. Transfer the mixture to your large baking dish and refrigerate until set completely before serving.

Nutrition: Calories: 72; Fat: 0g; Carbs: 16.1g; Protein: 2.2g

---

Almond Butter Banana Cream

 Prep Time: 5 minutes + chilling time   Cooking Time: 0 minutes   Servings: 6

INGREDIENTS

2 tsp vanilla extract
4 frozen bananas, chunks
½ cup non-dairy milk, unsweetened
½ cup almond butter

DIRECTIONS

1. Add the frozen bananas plus non-dairy milk to your food processor. Process them at low until bananas are creamy.
2. Add the almond butter plus vanilla extract to your food processor and process on low until blended. Add the banana mixture and pulse until evenly distributed.
3. Transfer to a dish and place in the freezer for 5-6 hours or overnight for a scoop-friendly nice cream.

Nutrition: Calories: 205; Fat: 12g; Carbs: 22g; Protein: 6g

Grape Gelatin

 Prep Time: 10 minutes

 Cooking Time: 0 minutes

 Servings: 8

INGREDIENTS

1 tbsp grass-fed gelatin powder
¼ cup cold filtered water
¼ cup hot water
1 cup fresh grape juice

DIRECTIONS

1. Soak the gelatin in cold water in your bowl. Set aside for about 5 minutes. Add the hot water and mix well. Set aside for about 1-2 minutes.
2. Add the grape juice and mix well. Divide into serving bowls and refrigerate until set completely before serving.

Nutrition: Calories: 17; Fat: 0g; Carbs: 3.7g; Protein: 0.69g

---

Strawberry Greek Yogurt Whip

 Prep Time: 10 minutes

 Cooking Time: 0 minutes

 Servings: 1

INGREDIENTS

no-calorie sweetener, to taste
3 fresh strawberries
2 tbsp light whipped topping
1/2 cup Greek yogurt, no-fat

DIRECTIONS

1. Coarsely mash the strawberries in a bowl and mix with yogurt and sweetener.
2. Fold the whipping topping and serve cold.

Nutrition: Calories 24; Carbs 3g; Fat 1g; Protein 8g

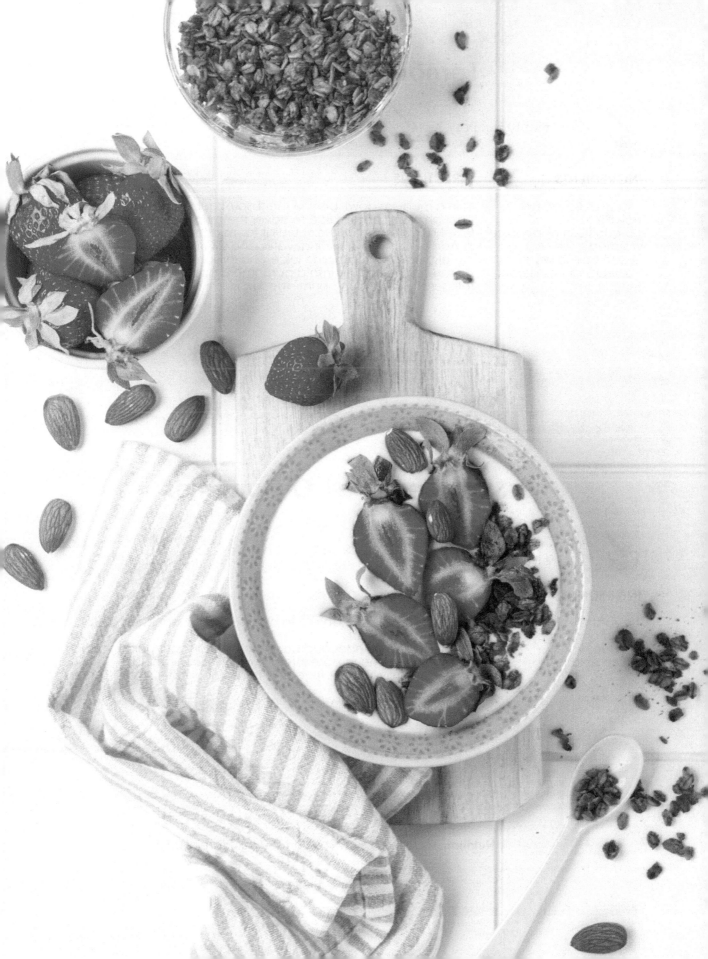

Lemony Apple Gelatin

 Prep Time: 10 minutes   Cooking Time: 0 minutes   Servings: 6

INGREDIENTS

1 tbsp grass-fed gelatin powder
1¾ cup fresh apple juice, warmed
¼ cup boiling water
1-2 drops of fresh lemon juice

DIRECTIONS

1. In a medium bowl, pour in the tbsp of gelatin powder. Add just enough warm apple juice to cover the gelatin and stir well.
2. Set aside for 3 minutes or until it forms a thick syrup.
3. Add ¼ cup of the boiling water and stir until gelatin is dissolved completely. Add the remaining juice and lemon juice and stir well.
4. Transfer the mixture into a parchment paper-lined baking dish and refrigerate for 2 hours or until the top is firm before serving.

Nutrition: Calories: 36; Fat: 0g; Carbs: 8.16g; Protein: 1g

Strawberry Jell-O Gummies

 Prep Time: 10 minutes + chilling time   Cooking Time: 5 minutes   Servings: 20-40 mini gummies

INGREDIENTS

1 cup strawberries, hulled and chopped
3/4 cup water
2 tbsp gelatin

DIRECTIONS

1. Bring your water and berries to a boil on high heat, then quickly remove them from the heat.
2. Transfer to the blender and pulse well. Add in your gelatin and pulse once more. Pour the mixture into a gummy silicone mold.
3. Place on a tray in the refrigerator to set for about 4 hours. Serve!

Nutrition: Calories: 4; Fat: 0g; Carbs: 0.5g; Protein: 0.6g

Lemon Gelatin

 Prep Time: 10 minutes + chilling time

 Cooking Time: 0 minutes

 Servings: 2

INGREDIENTS

3 tbsp powdered gelatin
1½ cup stevia
1 1/2 cups boiling water
3 cups cold water
1 1/8 cups lemon juice
1/2 tsp lemon zest

DIRECTIONS

1. Combine the gelatin and room temperature water, stirring until fully dissolved. Stir in hot water, then leave to rest for about 2 minutes.
2. Add all the remaining fixings and stir until combined.
3. Transfer to your containers, then place on a tray in the refrigerator to set for about 4 hours. Serve!

Nutrition: Calories: 66; Fat: 0.3g; Carbs: 135.6g; Protein: 9.4g

---

Cinnamon Tea Jelly

 Prep Time: 10 minutes + chilling time

 Cooking Time: 0 minutes

 Servings: 2

INGREDIENTS

1 cup hot herbal tea
1 cup room temperature water
2 tsp gelatin
1/3 cup stevia

DIRECTIONS

1. Combine your gelatin and room temperature water, stirring until fully dissolved. Stir in the herbal tea, then leave to rest for about 2 minutes.
2. Add the gelatin and stir until combined. Transfer to your containers, then place on a tray in the refrigerator to set for about 4 hours. Serve!
3.

Nutrition: Calories: 113; Fat: 0g; Carbs: 28.4g; Protein: 2.2g

Single Serve Baked Ricotta

 Prep Time: 10 minutes   Cooking Time: 20 minutes   Servings: 1

INGREDIENTS

1/7 cup low-fat cheese
salt and pepper, to taste
3 oz low-fat ricotta
1 tsp fresh basil, chop-
ped
1/8 tsp garlic powder

DIRECTIONS

1. Let the oven preheat to 350°F. Oil spray 1 ramekin and place on a baking tray.
2. In a bowl, mix all the ingredients. Transfer to the ramekin and bake for 15-20 minutes. Serve!

Nutrition: Calories 144; Carbs 5g; Fat 8g; Protein 12g

Honeydew Mint Popsicles

 Prep Time: 10 minutes +
freezing time   Cooking Time: 0 minutes   Servings: 10
popsicles

INGREDIENTS

½ honeydew melon,
peeled, seeded &
cubed
1/3 cup granulated
stevia
10 mint leaves
1 tbsp lime juice
6 oz water

DIRECTIONS

1. Blend all the fixings into your blender until smooth. Set a fine-mesh strainer in a bowl, and strain the blended mixture.
2. Press the pulp to extract all possible liquid, then discard the pulp. Pour your juice into your ice-pop molds, filling each three-quarter of the way.
3. Add in your ice pop sticks, then set to freeze for at least 5 hours or until solid. Serve.

Nutrition: Calories: 35; Fat: 0g; Carbs: 9g; Protein: 0.1g

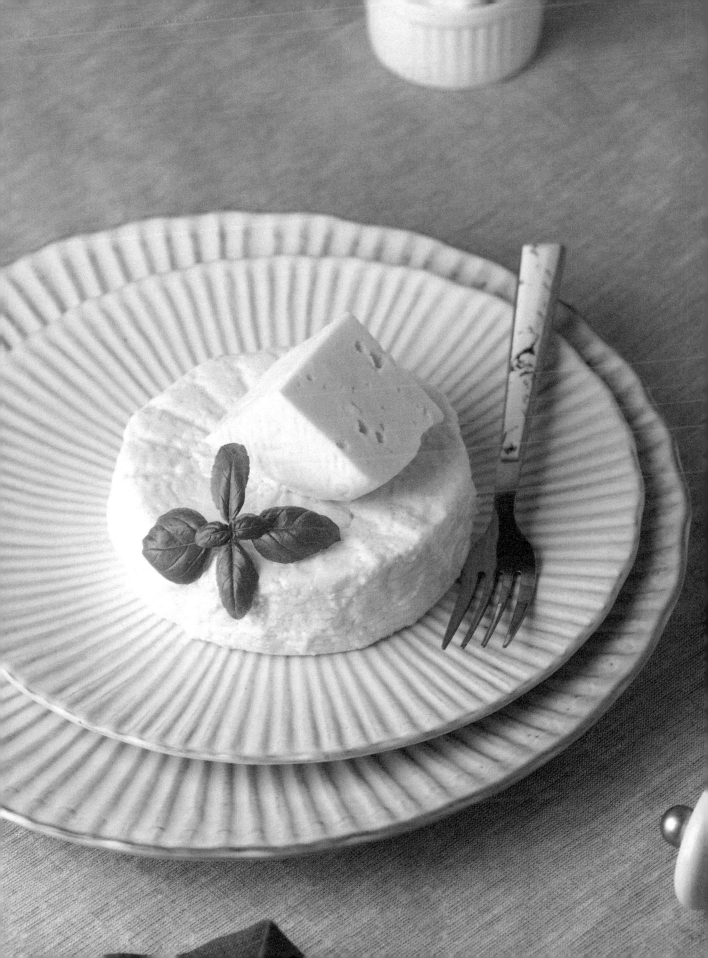

Tangerine Gelatin

 Prep Time: 10 minutes

 Cooking Time: 0 minutes

 Servings: 4

INGREDIENTS

1 tbsp Grass-fed tangerine gelatin powder
2 ¼ cups Boiling water

DIRECTIONS

1. Add the gelatin and boiling water to a large bowl and stir until dissolved completely.
2. Divide into serving bowls and refrigerate until set completely before serving.

Nutrition: Calories: 13; Fat: 0g; Carbs: 0.4g; Protein: 2.8g

Strawberry Watermelon Pops

 Prep Time: 10 minutes + freezing time

 Cooking Time: 0 minutes

 Servings: 12 pops

INGREDIENTS

2 cups watermelon, seeds removed and cubed
2 cups strawberries, fresh or frozen, quartered
¼ cup strawberry-flavored protein powder: whey isolate

DIRECTIONS

1. Place all fixings in a container of an electric blender. Cover and mix it until smooth.
2. Put it into popsicle molds and freeze them until popsicles are solid frozen for about six hours. Serve and enjoy!

Nutrition: Calories: 28; Fat: 0g; Carbs: 4g; Protein: 2.5g

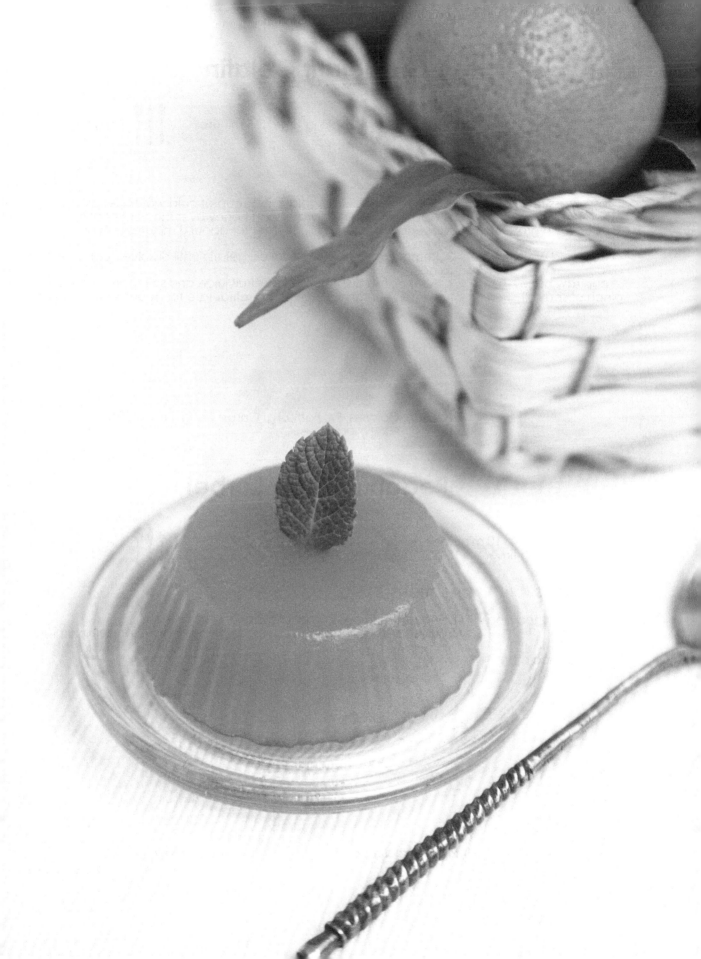

Grapefruit Gelatin

 Prep Time: 10 minutes + chilling time

 Cooking Time: 3-5 minutes

 Servings: 4

INGREDIENTS

1 tbsp grass-fed gelatin powder
1¼ cup fresh grapefruit juice
¾ cup cold water, divided
¼ cup raw honey
pinch of sea salt

DIRECTIONS

1. In a bowl, soak the gelatin in ¼ cup of cold water. Set aside.
2. Add the remaining water and honey over medium heat in your small saucepan and let it boil. Simmer for about 3 minutes until honey is dissolved completely.
3. Remove and stir in the soaked gelatin until dissolved completely. Set aside.
4. After cooling, stir in the grapefruit juice and salt. Transfer the mixture into your serving bowls and refrigerate for about 4 hours or until set.

Nutrition: Calories: 94; Fat: 0.1g; Carbs: 23.3g; Protein: 2g

---

Peach Mango Sorbet

 Prep Time: 10 minutes + freezing time

 Cooking Time: 0 minutes

 Servings: 2

INGREDIENTS

1½ cups canned peaches
3-4 tbsp stevia
1 cup canned mangoes/cherries

DIRECTIONS

1. Blend all the fixings in your blender until smooth
2. Transfer to your container, cover, and keep in your freezer overnight.

Nutrition: Calories: 81; Fat: 0.1g; Carbs: 21.3g; Protein: 0.6g

28- Day Meal Plan

	Breakfast	Lunch	Dinner	Snacks/Dessert
Day 1	Lemony Grape Juice	Carrot Potato Soup	Pumpkin Carrot Soup	Maple Orange Gelatin
Day 2	Apple Cider Water	Pumpkin Chicken Soup	Pureed Harvest Vegetable Chicken	Strawberry Watermelon Pops
Day 3	Papaya Carrot Smoothie	Pureed Refried Beans	Lettuce And Spinach Soup	Tangerine Gelatin
Day 4	Lemony Black Tea	Pureed Classic Egg Salad	Pureed Potato and Cheddar Mash	Peach Mango Sorbet
Day 5	Vanilla Apple Pie Shake	Clear Pumpkin Broth	Pureed Butternut Squash	Grapefruit Gelatin
Day 6	Citrus Sports Drink	Lettuce Cucumber Soup	Beef and Butternut Squash Stew	Cinnamon Tea Jelly
Day 7	Blueberry Green Tea	Chicken Carrot Broth	Ground Pork Sloppy Joe	Lemon Gelatin
Day 8	Fresh Mango Smoothie	Pureed Tuna-Avocado Salad	White Bean Soup	Honeydew Mint Popsicles
Day 9	No Pulp Orange Juice	Egg Whites	Beef Veggie Soup	Almond Butter Banana Cream
Day 10	Celery Apple Juice	Pureed Buffalo Ranch Chicken	Pureed Chimichurri Chicken	Single Serve Baked Ricotta

Day 11	Chilled Mint Green Tea	Pureed Turkey Tacos with Refried Beans	Mushroom Veggie Soup	Strawberry Jell-O Gummies
Day 12	Pineapple Mint Juice	Pureed Sweet Potato	Pureed Cheesy Cauliflower	Lemony Apple Gelatin
Day 13	Orange Green Tea	Pureed Lemon Garlic Salmon	Pureed Banana, Tofu & Pear	Strawberry Peach Pops
Day 14	Cucumber Cantaloupe Juice	Swede Soup	Pureed Chicken & Sweet Potato	Peach Gelatin
Day 15	Citrus Green Tea	Butternut Squash Curry Soup	Mexican Egg Puree	Strawberry Greek Yogurt Whip
Day 16	Applesauce-Avocado Smoothie	Red Lentil Mash	Pureed Caribbean Pork	Grape Gelatin
Day 17	Apple-Cinnamon Tea	Vegetable Broth	Pureed Cheeseburgers	Blackberry-Rose Ice Pops
Day 18	Cranberry Honey Juice	Pureed Italian Chicken	Creamy Cauliflower Soup	Easy Egg Custard
Day 19	Sage Rosemary Tea	Pureed Ricotta & White Bean	Pureed Chili	Low Fat Panna Cotta
Day 20	Turmeric Lemon & Ginger Tea	Creamy Shrimp Scampi	Light Tomato Soup	Strawberry Lemon Jell-O

Day 21	Vanilla Bean Probiotic Shake	Root Vegetable Soup	Pureed Chicken Breast Salad	Honey Lemonade Popsicles
Day 22	Refreshing Strawberry Smoothie	Cauliflower Tofu Puree	Pureed Mediterranean Chicken	Pumpkin Fluff
Day 23	Carrot Orange Juice	Pureed Chicken with Black Bean Mole	Pureed Rosemary Chicken with Blue Cheese	Orange Sugar-Free Gelatin
Day 24	Cantaloupe-Mix Smoothie	Pureed Roasted Carrot	Pureed Ginger Garlic Tofu	Cranberry-Kombucha Jell-O
Day 25	Spiced Ginger Tea	Creamy Carrot and Ginger Soup	Pureed Moroccan Fish	Maple Orange Gelatin
Day 26	Lemony Grape Juice	Carrot Potato Soup	Pureed Sesame Tuna Salad	Strawberry Watermelon Pops
Day 27	Apple Cider Water	Pumpkin Chicken Soup	Pumpkin Carrot Soup	Tangerine Gelatin
Day 28	Papaya Carrot Smoothie	Pureed Refried Beans	Pureed Harvest Vegetable Chicken	Peach Mango Sorbet

Cooking Conversion Chart

Volume Equivalent (Liquid)

US STANDARD	US STANDARD (OUNCES)	METRIC (APPROXIMATE)
2 tablespoons	1 fl. oz.	30 mL
¼ cup	2 fl. oz.	60 mL
½ cup	4 fl. oz.	120 mL
1 cup	8 fl. oz.	240 mL
1½ cups	12 fl. oz.	355 mL
2 cups or 1 pint	16 fl. oz.	475 mL
4 cups or 1 quart	32 fl. oz.	1 L
1 gallon	128 fl. oz.	4 L

Oven Temperature

FAHRENHEIT (F)	CELSIUS (C) (APPROXIMATE)
250	120
300	150
325	165
350	180
375	190
400	200
425	220
450	230

Volume Equivalent (Dry)

US STANDARD	METRIC (APPROXIMATE)
⅛ teaspoon	0.5 mL
¼ teaspoon	1 mL
½ teaspoon	2 mL
¾ teaspoon	4 mL
1 teaspoon	5 mL
1 tablespoon	15 mL
¼ cup	59 mL
⅓ cup	79 mL
½ cup	118 mL
⅔ cup	156 mL
¾ cup	177 mL
1 cup	235 mL
2 cups or 1 pint	475 mL
3 cups	700 mL
4 cups or 1 quart	1 L
½ gallon	2 L
1 gallon	4 L

Wheight Equivalent

US STANDARD	METRIC (APPROXIMATE)
½ ounce	15 g
1 ounce	30 g
2 ounces	60 g
4 ounces	115 g
8 ounces	225 g
12 ounces	340 g
16 ounces or 1 pound	455 g

Conclusion

Anyone can have dysphagia at any age, but it is most common in older adults. It occurs when there is a problem with any part of the process of swallowing. Dysphagia can be temporary or ongoing. It can be caused by a number of things, including a physical blockage, damage to the nerves or muscles involved in swallowing, or an underlying medical condition.

If you or you know someone who is struggling with dysphagia, a specific diet may be recommended by a medical professional. A dysphagia diet is a diet that is designed to make eating and drinking easier for people who have trouble swallowing. The diet usually contains fewer calories and more fluids than a regular diet. The goal is to keep the person's body hydrated and help them get the nutrients they need without having to swallow large chunks of food.

There are a number of different types of dysphagia diets, but all of them involve eating soft foods that are easy to chew and swallow. A lot of the foods on a dysphagia diet are protein- and fiber-rich, which is why many people find them satisfying. The 28-day meal plan included with this book provides recommendations with our 100 delicious and nourishing soft-food recipes to make meal planning a breeze.

If you decide to try a dysphagia diet, be sure to consult with a doctor or nutritionist to make sure it's the right fit for you.

Made in United States
Orlando, FL
14 December 2024